LAW, CRIME AND LAW ENFORCEMENT

LISTENING TO THEIR VOICES OF BRAVERY AND HEROISM

EXPLORING THE AFTERMATH OF OFFICERS' LOSS AND TRAUMA IN THE LINE OF DUTY

LAW, CRIME AND LAW ENFORCEMENT

Additional books in this series can be found on Nova's website under the Series tab.

Additional e-books in this series can be found on Nova's website under the eBooks tab.

LAW, CRIME AND LAW ENFORCEMENT

LISTENING TO THEIR VOICES OF BRAVERY AND HEROISM

EXPLORING THE AFTERMATH OF OFFICERS' LOSS AND TRAUMA IN THE LINE OF DUTY

KONSTANTINOS PAPAZOGLOU
EDITOR

NOVINKA

New York

NOTICE TO THE READER

Library of Congress Cataloging-in-Publication Data

ISBN: 978-1-53610-048-8

Published by Nova Science Publishers, Inc. † New York

This book is dedicated to:

My spouse – Irene – for her remarkable patience, love, and encouragement to fulfill my academic and professional goals

The memory of my grandfather – Athanasius - (World War I refugee and World War II Veteran) and my grandmother – Dominique – (World War I refugee) who have always been missed since they passed. They instilled in my life precious values (perseverance, pride, forgiveness, and justice) and inspired me to support those who suffer in life with kindness, caring, and altruism

The memory of all law enforcement officers who sacrificed their lives in the line of duty. May God rest them in peace and bless their families

September 29th, 2016
Toronto, Ontario, Canada

Konstantinos Papazoglou
Psychology Doctoral (PhD) Candidate in Clinical – Forensic area
University of Toronto – Vanier Scholar;
Police Captain (former)
Hellenic National Police – European Police College

Contents

Prologue

The Unique Nature of Police Work: Oscillating between Crime Fighting and Victim Support

Most people, if asked about police work, would probably suggest that police work is mainly focused on crime investigations, patrol, or arrest of criminals. Nevertheless, the reality of what police work entails is more complex than many people may presume. Undeniably, police officers are often crime fighters and, as such, they are sworn and mandated to respond to virulent crimes (i.e., terrorism attacks, murders) and arrest the criminal(s). Notwithstanding, the other side of the coin, which is often ignored by many of us, is that police officers support victims of crimes (i.e., abused children, battered women) since they are often amongst the first responders present at the crime scene. For instance, when the mass school shooting occurred in Newtown, Connecticut, police officers were the first respondents at the scene first (Draznin, 2013). As a result, they were the ones holding the wounded children and providing them with first aid as well as psychological support. What many of us do not consider, is that police officers are exposed to a plethora of threatening – and potentially traumatic situations - over the course of their careers. Therefore, what makes police work unique is that police officers are expected to diligently maintain a dual role; that is, police officers often oscillate between in their roles as “crime fighters” and their roles as “social service workers.” Some police psychologists and scholars argue that police officers may encounter - not surprisingly - hundreds of adverse events during their career.

Psychological Trauma and Resilience Among Police Officers

Psychological trauma refers to any sudden, uncontrollable, and disruptive incident that negatively affects one's physical, emotional, behavioral, and cognitive processes, and consequently, that may beget various forms of psychopathology (i.e., post-traumatic stress reactivity, major depression) (Van der Kolk, 2003). The origin of term "trauma" can be traced back to the Greek term "τραύμα" which literally means "to wound." (Oxford Dictionary, 2015). In the area of psychological trauma, the etymology of the verb "to wound" insinuates the "psychological wounds" that may emanate from exposure to any traumatic incident. Psychological research of the impact of trauma to police officers has shown that experience of trauma may be debilitating for police officers' physical (i.e., high blood pressure, cardiovascular diseases) and psychological health (i.e., anxiety disorder, depression) over the course of their careers (Miller, 2000; Stephens, Long, & Miller, 1997; Violanti et al., 2006). Furthermore, exposure to traumatic incidents may adversely affect police officers' behavior (i.e., impatience, anger outbursts), cognitive processes (i.e., memory, information processing), and emotional reactivity to daily life (i.e., sadness, feeling like a failure) (Andersen, Papazoglou, Arnetz, & Collins, 2015). As aforementioned, police trauma is cumulative, long-term, and complex on the grounds that police officers – on a regular basis – experience multiple potentially traumatic incidents over the course of their careers (Papazoglou, 2013). The complexity of police trauma refers to the fact that officers may experience trauma directly (i.e., loss of a partner) or indirectly (i.e., ask a victim of abuse to describe what happened). In police work, trauma is often experienced with some or all of our human senses. For instance, a life-threatening situation (i.e., shooting) experienced by a police officer in the line of duty, may involve the following senses: visual (officer was at the incident), auditory (officer listened to the shooting sounds), olfactory (officer smelt the smoke of the firing bullet), and touch (officer held the weapon during the incident). Another parameter that needs to be considered akin to police trauma is that police officers have their own distinct culture comprised of a unique framework of values, tenets, attitudes, and lingo (Crank & Crank, 2014; Paoline, 2003). Analytically, police culture instills in its members the sense of group cohesiveness and brotherhood/sisterhood-like loyalty, in connection to crime fighting and officer's own bodily survival on the street. Significantly, another major component of police culture is the salient role of teamwork and reciprocity in facing adversities in the line of duty.

Nonetheless, human beings have the capacity to not only survive the aftermath of trauma but also to recover (or else adapt) and thrive in their post-trauma lives (Bonanno, 2004, 2005). In the police field, although police officers seem to experience more trauma-related psychological symptoms compared to the general population, research has indicated that police officers are significantly more resilient in the face of adversities, and better armored to resolve traumatic situations compared to the general public (Galatzer-Levy et al., 2013; Marmar et al., 2006; Miller, 2000).

CURRENT PROJECT

In this book we present the case reports of law enforcement officers vis-à-vis their unique experiences of trauma and loss in the line of duty. Further, this project's case reports illustrate the impact of trauma and loss on our participants' health as well as on their personal and professional lives. We also aimed to explore the strengths and coping mechanisms that helped our participants' adapt in the aftermath of their traumatic experiences. Various questions subsequently emerged in response to participants' testimonials. For example: What made our participants resilient? What were their recommendations for other police officers and health professionals? All the cases illustrated in this project have been extensively covered in public and social medial nationally and internationally. In this project we disguised our participants' personal information in order to protect their personal identities. Nevertheless, we retained all other information provided by our participants allowing the readers to read of their stories of bravery and heroism. Analytically, the case reports analyzed and discussed in this project are as follows:

Chapter 1. Facing the Perpetrator Again. Officers' Re-Traumatization when Testifying duringCriminal Trials: An Unexplored Issue. This chapter presents the experience of two Southern European police officers, through interview, who were shot multiple times and seriously wounded by a terrorist (armed anarchist). Following their physical recovery they then had to testify in court while exposed to the terrorist's death threats and hate speech, which was allowed to be voiced in the courtroom.

Chapter 2. Police Officers being held Hostages on a Peacekeeping Mission: Exploring a Unique Form of Police Trauma. In this chapter, we present the case of two police officers from a Nordic country who were deployed on a UN peacekeeping mission during the war in former Yugoslavia. Police officers in this case were kept as hostages by a group of armed guerrillas.

Chapter 3. Once "Blue" Always "Blue": A Law Enforcement Professional Thwarts Mass Shooting in a Public Place. This chapter illustrates the case of a US law enforcement professional who effectively stopped a mass shooter in a religious assembly right after he started shooting civilians. Kathy (pseudonym) faced and stopped the mass shooter using her weapon saving the lives of thousands of people.

Chapter 4. Exploring the Experiences of Police Officers who Deadly Shot Suspects in the Line of Duty. Over the last years, there has been great controversy surrounding police officers using weapons on unarmed civilians. However, there is a lack of research to explore the consequences that these officers experience following these events. In the present chapter, we present the case of two officers from North America (US and Canada) who shot and killed suspects who they - mistakenly - believed to be armed. These officers shared with us the details of their incidents and the bureaucratic procedures that followed the shooting events.

Chapter 5. Exploring SWAT Officers' Experiences of Trauma and Resilience. SWAT team officers are trained in the use of sophisticated equipment and have advanced tactical knowledge to combat high-risk critical situations. Nevertheless, traumatic experiences are often embedded in SWAT team officers' missions. In this chapter, we explore the life-threatening cases experienced by three SWAT team officers from a Nordic country.

METHODOLOGY: PROCEDURES AND DATA ANALYSIS

Research that explores the psychological effects of unprecedented trauma and loss in the line of duty is limited. Police officers who have survived life-threatening situations are often skeptical to share their experiences with an "outsider" to police culture. Nevertheless, our background (police and military) helped us approach several such police officers, who subsequently accepted our invitation to share their stories of how they survived life-threatening situations. The interviews occurred in places that were preferred by the participants; hence, participants' police units, family houses, and therapists' offices were chosen as places where the interviews would take place. The interviews lasted 3 hours on average. Written informed consent for participants in this project was obtained at the outset of the interview. In most of the cases, participants were informed that their department's clinical psychologist was aware of their interview, and that s/he was available to provide psychological support, if needed. Alternatively, in some other cases discussed in this project, participants were allowed - and preferred - to refer to their own clinician in the case that they had been in psychotherapy or psychiatric medical treatment before their participation in the current study.

We conducted in-depth and semi-structured interviews with open-ended questions. Consequently, we were able to maintain flexible, spontaneous, and natural conversations which ultimately allowed participants to feel comfortable enough to share their experiences with us. We conducted one-on-one interviews and the sessions were voice recorded and transcribed by our research assistants. In order to validate our findings, we followed Denzin's (1989) approach for illuminating the phenomenon in a thickly contextualized manner, so as to reveal interactional features of the police officers' experience. To further validate the findings, an inter-coder agreement was reached by the authors. We also examined the transcripts numerous times doing several readings of the narratives to identify recurring themes. Audio files of interviews and their corresponding field notes, in addition to data analysis drafts, were maintained for peer review and to re-check the validity of the findings. Taking into account the aims of this project we emphasized our coding based on officers' survival skills during a life-threatening situation, strengths and coping skills during and after the traumatic incident, trauma-related symptomatology, and the role of others (i.e., family, friends, colleagues, organization) in the aftermath of trauma. The study was approved by the Research Ethics Board at the University of Toronto.

References

Andersen, J.P., Papazoglou, K., Arnetz, B.B., & Collins, P.I. (2015). Mental Preparedness as a Pathway to Police Resilience and Optimal Functioning in the Line of Duty. *International Journal of Emergency Mental Health, 17*(3), 624-627.

Bonanno, G. A. (2004). Loss, trauma, and human resilience: have we underestimated the human capacity to thrive after extremely aversive events? *American psychologist, 59*(1), 20-28.

Bonanno, G. A. (2005). Resilience in the face of potential trauma. *Current directions in psychological science*, *14*(3), 135-138.

Crank, J., & Crank, J. P. (2014). *Understanding police culture*. New York, NY: Routledge.

Denzin, R.K. (1989). *Interpretive biography*. Newbury Park, CA: Sage.

Draznin, H. (2013). Report supports police report time to Newtown shooting. CNN Justice. Retrieved from: http://www.cnn.com/2013/12/06/justice/newtown-police-response-school-shooting/.

Galatzer-Levy, I. R., Brown, A. D., Henn-Haase, C., Metzler, T. J., Neylan, T. C., & Marmar, C. R. (2013). Positive and negative emotion prospectively predict trajectories of resilience and distress among high-exposure police officers. *Emotion*, *13*(3), 545.

Marmar, C. R., McCaslin, S. E., Metzler, T. J., Best, S., Weiss, D. S., Fagan, J., & Neylan, T. (2006). Predictors of posttraumatic stress in police and other first responders. *Annals of the New York Academy of Sciences*, *1071*(1), 1-18.

Miller, L. (2000). Law enforcement traumatic stress: Clinical syndromes and intervention strategies. *Trauma Response*, *6*(1), 15-20.

Oxford English Online Dictionary (September, 2015). Retrieved from: www.oed.com

Paoline, E. A. (2003). Taking stock: Toward a richer understanding of police culture. *Journal of criminal justice*, *31*(3), 199-214.

Papazoglou, K. (2013). Conceptualizing Police Complex Spiral Trauma and its applications in the police field. *Traumatology*, *19*(3), 196-209.

Stephens, C., Long, N., & Miller, I. (1997). The impact of trauma and social support on posttraumatic stress disorder: A study of New Zealand police officers. *Journal of Criminal Justice*, *25*(4), 303-314.

Van der Kolk, B. A. (2003). *Psychological Trauma*. Washington, DC: American Psychiatric Publishing.

Violanti, J. M., Burchfiel, C. M., Miller, D. B., Andrew, M. E., Dorn, J., Wactawski-Wende, J., & Trevisan, M. (2006). The buffalo cardio-metabolic occupational police stress (BCOPS) pilot study: methods and participant characteristics. *Annals of epidemiology*, *16*(2), 148-156.

In: Listening to their Voices of Bravery
Editor: Konstantinos Papazoglou
ISBN: 978-1-53610-048-8

Chapter 1

FACING THE PERPETRATOR AGAIN. OFFICERS' RE-TRAUMATIZATION WHEN TESTIFYING DURING CRIMINAL TRIALS: AN UNEXPLORED ISSUE

Konstantinos Papazoglou* and Shelly-Anne Li†
University of Toronto, ON, Canada

INTRODUCTION

Police officers are often exposed to multiple critical incidents (e.g., domestic violence, terrorist attacks, life-threatening situations) over the course of their careers (Kingshott, Bailey, & Wolfe, 2004). This means that trauma experienced by officers is often prolonged, complex, and cumulative over the course of police career (Papazoglou, 2013). Moreover, repeated exposure to adverse incidents increases risks for both mental (Hall et al., 2010) and physical health (Andersen et al., 2010). Other researchers (Huddleston, Stephens, & Paton, 2007) argue that the role of the organization often contributes to the deterioration of officers' health, because work-related stress

* Psychology PhD Candidate in Clinical-Forensic area, Vanier Scholar; Police Captain (former) Police Academy, Hellenic National Police and European Police College.
† PhD Candidate in Health Systems Research, University of Toronto, ON, Canada

within the organization is often more frequent than adverse events experienced on the street.

The unique nature of police work has led to the development of a distinct "police culture," one that provides officers with a sense of belonging and cohesiveness and is characterized by certain rules, traditions, and jargon (Kingshott, Bailey, & Wolfe, 2004). Within this culture, exposure to adversities is considered to be part of the job, and hence, has traditionally not been recognized as a risk factor for health problems over time (Rudofossi, 2007). However, researchers in the field of trauma and loss have focused on police officers' traumatic deaths or serious injuries in the line of duty, the way officers experience life-threatening situations, and the impact of such incidents in their lives (Sugimoto & Oltjenbruns, 2001). In addition, Komarovskaya and colleagues (2011) studied officers' experiences with killing or seriously injuring someone in the line of duty, and the negative impact of such experiences on the officer's health and life.

Our Rationale - Why a Case Report?

Trauma literature includes studies that emphasize the experiences of victims/survivors (e.g., rape crimes) who have to testify in court (Orth & Maercker, 2004). Despite the fact that police work is demanding and dangerous, similar experiences of police officers have yet to be studied. Research exploring the experience of officers who are exposed to life-threatening incidents and are then expected to go to trial and testify about their experience is rare. These officers are often required to face the perpetrators in court, with potentially very negative effects. We present the case of two operational police officers who were seriously wounded in the line of duty by a terrorist, and who afterwards had to testify of their experiences in court, facing the perpetrator. What makes their case even more unique is that during the day of the trial, they experienced threats and hateful speech from the other members of the same terrorist group. The two officers, Evans and Victor (pseudonyms), stated that "after the incident per se, the trial was like a second round, like a psychological war. In other words, we experienced the real fire. Now we are going to experience the 'psychological fire.' " Our goal is to pose and answer the following questions that have not previously been addressed in trauma literature: What was the experience of the two officers exposed to cumulative trauma during these two critical incidents? What helped the two officers cope in the aftermath of the trauma (line of duty) and re-traumatization (trial)? We attempt to identify the unique coping mechanisms and personal strengths that helped them survive an imminent confrontation with death, and handle the re-experience of the trauma during the trial. We hope that findings from our case report will open further research and discussion about police officers' experience of trauma and re-traumatization when they are mandated to testify in court.

What Happened?

It was the fall of 2009 when the two officers, Evans and Victor, were patrolling an area of a metropolitan city. The two officers received a call on their radio that a grocery store owner noticed a person wandering around for at least two hours in the park across from his grocery store. The two officers responded to the call, a routine security check, similar to calls they had answered a hundred times before during their careers. When the officers arrived, the person turned his back to them and started running. They ran after him. When Victor was close to catching up to him, the perpetrator took out his weapon and shot at him twice. Then, the offender turned and shot at Evans several times. Evans and Victor were not able to react and defend themselves, since the first bullets hit vital parts of their bodies. While they were bleeding on the ground, the offender kept shooting at them multiple times, until he emptied a whole round of ammunition. The officers were hospitalized for three months. The doctors stated that they both survived almost miraculously. The offender was soon arrested after the incident and police reported that he was a member of one of the most vicious terrorist groups (armed anarchists), with a history of having repeatedly attacked police officers. In the spring of 2010, Evans and Victor were asked to testify about the incident in court. Security forces guarded the court and the area around it. However, some of the terrorist group members and relatives of the terrorist were in the courtroom, and the spaces around the courtroom (e.g., hall entrance to the court). During the trial, the two officers, once again, met with their perpetrator, who openly stated to the judges and jurors that he was proud of what he did, and that he regretted not having killed the officers. Although the terrorist was arrested and charged with life-long incarceration, his actions were considered, by his fellow terrorists, to be an "act of bravery." The terrorist group continues to uphold the oath that injuring or killing police officers, regardless of the outcome, is an "act of bravery." During the trial, and while the two officers were waiting at the entrance hall, members of the terrorist group and family members of the terrorist approached them with threats, curses, and malicious gestures.

Evans and Victor described what happened to them as follows:

> "The first time I was shocked because of the incident ... not because I got shot ... but ... I felt the hatred of those who shot me ... his aim to kill me ... you think you are going to die.... I was in the hospital and they were coming to visit me there, and I was thinking and I was telling them 'you know what? he wanted to kill me' I really believe that ... I felt his hatred. After the incident ... the worst thing that you face is the trial ... and ... they had ... the support from a group of people with the same ideology who were in the court.... It was very difficult because you feel isolated ... they come close to you and they whisper ... and in general they make you feel like it is all your fault for risking your life to maintain peace and order, and for fighting to protect the common welfare of the people ... you feel like a piece of garbage...."

METHODS

Evans and Victor (pseudonyms) chose to participate in the interview with the researchers about their experiences. The interview took place in their police unit, located on the outskirts of their city. They had asked for the interviewer to meet in the late afternoon, after their shift, to ensure a quiet and undisturbed environment. The room had a long rectangular table with a few chairs, and two large windows with a view of the mountains. The two officers were dressed casually - both wore jeans and long-sleeve shirts and had their cell phones turned off prior to beginning of the interview. They were sitting next to each other (around the corner of the table), and the interviewer was sitting across from them. Evans and Victor were open and willing to share their experiences, provided that their personal identities would not be disclosed. They insisted on being interviewed together because they posited that being together made them feel safer. The officers stated that they were eager to make researchers, clinicians, and students, aware of the risks and adversities of police work. Further, they hoped that by sharing their experiences, the information would motivate changes to policies within police departments related to providing adequate support to officers who have experienced such adversities.

Evans and Victor were both single men in their early forties of Southern European descent. They served as patrol officers in a metropolitan city for over ten years. They were patrolling together for 3 years before the incident occurred. The research participants insisted on conducting the interview to recount the events and experiences related to the traumatic incident. The two officers found the interview distressing but manageable and possible helpful since they had the opportunity to "have their voices heard."

FINDINGS

The Officers' View of the Adverse Incidents

Facing Death

During the event, the two officers commented "everything happened so fast." They also made clear that what happened to them was something unpredictable, since the perpetrator surprised them with "a very ... short ... ill-prepared ambush." They commented that they had some "black spots" in their attempt to recall details of the incident, and they also mentioned that they remembered pictures of the incident like "watching a movie." Evans mentioned that he could see general figures around him in a dark background and he was not able to distinguish details. Evans and Victor contend that their situation was even more complicated since they had to make a decision on how they needed to react to the perpetrator's shooting at them: "I have to use my weapon ... Where do you shoot? ... Who is shooting you? ... Where is your partner? ... Where are the offenders?....". Even though the incident lasted only seconds, it gave the officers the sense that it lasted for a much longer time. Evans mentioned that when he was bleeding on the ground, he tried to focus his attention on something that would help him to stay awake. He commented: "I was somehow losing my consciousness, and I was trying to stay awake ... because I was afraid that if I became unconscious ... I would die ... I was trying again to get strength and focus on something that would keep me awake....." Evans and Victor had a sense that they were almost dead. They knew they had been wounded in vital parts of their body. Notwithstanding, the two officers referred to the fear they felt not only of dying, but of losing important people in their lives: "You are going to die and the first thing that you think of is your own people." Moreover, they referred to their fear of losing each other, and their eventual relief and gratitude when they realized that their partner was still alive: "You are happy because at some point you believed that you were losing them (family, police partner, friends)….I didn't lose him (partner) ….apparently he didn't lose me."

They are trying to find an explanation for what helped them during that moment when they both were bleeding on the ground. They expressed faith that something or someone intervened to ensure their survival. They commented: "Somebody might call it randomness, a religious person might say that God helped me ... it is the way you view things ... we literally survived and it was a matter of millimeters ... even doctors were surprised they could not believe how we survived....." In his attempt to give a possible explanation of what helped them, Victor said: "Whatever helped us I want to show my gratefulness, either this is God, or randomness, or whatever else....."

The Trial

Evans and Victor were exposed to a second traumatic situation, the trial, where they were obligated to recall the incident and to testify regarding what happened under oath. They both said: "After the incident ... the worst thing that you face is the trial ... the trial was like a second round, like a psychological war." They asked their family members not to show up for the trial. They wanted to protect them from the emotional pain they might have experienced, with the detailed recollection of the incidents, and presentation of evidence that was going to be processed in the trial. Therefore, they experienced a great deal of isolation. In their own words: "At that moment we were feeling that nobody is around to support and protect us ... police officers ... we were alone in a hall." Even though they risked their lives in the line of duty, they experienced worthlessness and humiliation by the terrorist group members who supported the terrorist, Evans and Victor described the psychological threat posed by the supporters of their perpetrator, as follows:

> "They humiliate you ... they curse you ... they call you names ... they come close to you and they whisper ... 'you are a cop you deserve to die ... you should have died.' None of this was heard by the judges. In general, they make you feel like a piece of garbage, you are nothing ... the value of life is ... nothing ... it is difficult ... to be in a place where you have to face this attitude…."

The mounting experience of isolation and worthlessness during the trial seemed to impose a sense of guilt upon the officers, who have been victimized emotionally at this time. Evans and Victor's apologetic attitude brings this out clearly: “we did not overly use our guns, even during the incident...we did not cause this ... we were attacked unexpectedly ... we didn't violate the law.”

The Perpetrator

Evans and Victor contended that the perpetrator was determined to kill them. They both felt the perpetrator’s hatred while he was shooting at them. They could not believe how somebody could do that to another human being, since the perpetrator did not try to escape, but kept shooting at them while they were bleeding on the ground. What further disappointed the two officers was that the perpetrator who displayed no remorse in the trial. Significantly, his act against them was considered an “act of valor” by the terrorist group members, and he himself was considered by them to be “a hero because he killed a cop.” This situation led Evans and Victor to adapt a tone of sarcasm during the trial as they recounted their experiences: “He (the perpetrator) goes to jail and everybody (his supporters) is there to be proud of their ‘brave’ boy who managed to shoot and wound a police officer who they wished would have died.”

Officers’ Symptoms in the Aftermath of the Life-Threating Incident

Reliving the Life-Threatening Incident

Evans and Victor mention that, almost daily, their minds were occupied with what happened to them. They tried to avoid the memories but could not escape reliving the event. Moreover, the re-experiencing of the incident by being required to face the perpetrator in court was an emotionally painful situation for them. Their minds were pre-occupied with the facing death incident. The repetitive reminder of the incident made them feel panicked and stuck. In particular, they felt sadness that they were not able to escape the attack. The two officers remarked:

> “I was recalling this incident in parts and many times ... in general though it is a painful experience, an experience that takes time to get out of the mind and ... whether you want to or not, you cannot avoid that ... it's very hard ... you were almost dead ... and there is no worse feeling than that ... you re-experience that, and the other people are asking you ‘are you ok?’ and you are telling them ‘yes I am fine ... I’ll be fine in a bit’ something like that.”

It seems, however, that as time passed by, they became better able to handle their "feeling stuck" symptoms and to control their re-experiencing of the event in their own ways. Nightmares were also pervasive in the lives of the two officers. They described their nightmares as recurring, haunting, and that such dreams made them feel sad and fearful. They stated that they consistently woke up in the middle of the night, only to realize that "it was just a bad dream ... fortunately, I survived ….." Victor and Evans mentioned that they had these "bad dreams" even when they were sitting with other people. They described their flashbacks as "something like a dream that was coming over and over again….."

The Connection between Mental and Physical Health

Evans and Victor talked about the connection between mental and physical health. They mentioned the fact that they are both physically well is very important for them. They were seriously wounded during the incident, and each of them was hospitalized for three months. Since then, they have physically recovered. A potential severe physical health issue (e.g., amputation) would have affected them psychologically. Evans stated that one of the main things that helped them feel psychologically better in the aftermath of their trauma was the fact that they recovered physically. He then commented: "If I had even one serious issue ... requiring amputation ... or been wounded to my joints and forced to walk with a limp, I believe I would have experienced much severe psychological issues ...."

Role of Others

Public Attention

The incident was in the local news for an extended period of time. Many people who knew the two officers, some out of curiosity, and others out of authentic interest, contacted them to ask about their health conditions and recovery. What made the two officers very angry was the attitude of some people who tried to tell them what they should have done in order to avoid this incident. Victor commented,

> "These people didn't know how the incident happened or they were trying to show us that they are smart ... they were telling us things that were not accurate about the incident ... nobody knows what happened ... except us who were there ... even us we have gaps in our memories...."

However, most of the people recognized their sacrifice and congratulated them. Evans and Victor stated: "You get their congratulations and their encouragement ... and they made you feel good."

The Role of the Organization

Evans reported that high-ranked managers tried to treat them well the first few months after the incident because it was in the local and national news for a long period of time. Evans suggests with sarcasm, that the high-ranked managers were more concerned about the incident because it was in the news than genuine concern for him and Victor. They stated that the high-ranked managers' interest about their case declined as time passed by and the case was not in the news anymore. Victor critiqued the role of the high-ranked managers saying that "many times, they didn't understand our situation ... they would say: 'we need to move on'.... and you see their ignorance." They also referred to the role of the supervisors who tried to take advantage of the officers' sacrifice "not necessarily in bad ways" but to show off that their guys were wounded ... " 'Look my officers are at risk, I need more personnel....' "

Psychologists of the police organization invited the two officers for psychological support, making it clear that they were welcome in their offices. Evans and Victor visited the psychologist of the organization two or three times after the incident in order "to see what they had to tell us....." Even though the psychologists told them that "their door was open" both officers eventually preferred not to "knock [at] their door." They contended that they could get over the impact of their adversities on their own, even if that way was harder for them.

Family and Friends' Concern

The officers' families and friends were critical in providing them with support and helping them in many ways to cope in the aftermath of their adverse experiences. Both Evans and Victor realized how their families suffered for what happened. For their families, the event "was something terrible....." Their families were often over-protective or worried whenever the two officers had symptoms related to the incident. Their families panicked that the officers might not recover from the impact of the incident. As a result, Evans and Victor often "pretended that [they were] fine" in order to appease their families with the illusion that they were doing well.

Lessons Learned after the Incidents

Evans and Victor attempted to comprehend the meaning of what they experienced ("lessons we learned") after the trial was finished. They stated that after a certain period of time, things went back to normal but that they learned to view certain things from a different perspective; above all, appreciating what they have. They also tried to change the way they view things around them. For instance, they try to "have laughs in their lives …. avoid being miserable in life and focus on having a good quality of life." Evans stated that emotional regulation and calmness helped him not to panic when he was encountering the perpetrator. He also stated that calmness helped him to "make the right decision ... because sometimes you need not to react in order to survive ... overall one needs to be able to remain calm." Victor re-assessed the impact of the incident saying to himself "fortunately I survived ... it's [the impact of the incident] less important to me."

Coping Mechanisms

Self-Reliance

Family members and friends became worried when they realized that the two officers still had issues related to the incident (e.g., nightmares, flashbacks). As a result, they showed their family members that they were doing better than they were, and not experiencing any issues related to the incident. While they had the public's attention, the public, as well as the police community, upheld expectations for the police officers to be strong and able to get over the impact of their trauma soon. Evans' words are quite powerful at this moment, and manifest the strength of the two officers to support themselves, as well as their families and friends. Evans remarked,

> "Whether you like it or not you have to overcome this ... to overcome the whole situation by the effort that you make to support your family, your siblings, when they come to visit you (in the hospital) they should not see you lying in bed ... and you should show them that you can stand on your own feet ... and not seeing you lying on the bed with the oxygen mask ... all this ... forces you to overcome this ... it's ourselves ... our own strength ... the strength inside you ... you need to support in your own way, those who support you, in order to make them feel better."

Role of Partner

The role of the partner was an integral part of the way the two officers coped in the aftermath of their traumatic experiences. The agony of Evans and Victor of having potentially lost each other when they were bleeding on the ground is clearly stated by both: "When the other patrol cars and paramedics came we were asking 'how is my partner?' and they were saying 'we don't know' because we were far from each other." They both stated that the experience would have been much harder for them if one of the two had died ("I don't want to even think about it….."). Afterwards, being in different wings of the hospital, since they were wounded in different parts of their bodies, they were not able to see each other. However, it was their demand to "be in the same room ... it couldn't have happened in a different way….." The strong bonds and the unity between the two seem to have been present since they first met. They reported: "We have gone through everything together ... even in the court we go together ... we never abandon each other in whatever happens." Victor reported that if one of them would have died, then the other would have blamed himself for doing something wrong. They remarked: "We were together giving advice and recommendations to each other ... we went through that together." The strength of unity and caring between the two partners became apparent in a powerful moment at the end of the interview, when Victor turned to his partner, Evans, and said: "I would like to say, in public, because I know that this interview will be presented in public to thank my partner...because he was there... every time we were in danger."

Solidarity in Police Culture

Evans and Victor received their colleagues' genuine empathy and emotional support. They have maintained trusted relationships with their colleagues at the same level with those between family members. Specifically, they reported that "the person who sits next to you in the patrol car is your brother, your friend, your father ... you should respect and always be there and support him/her." In addition, this sense of respect and support among officers is mutual since "s/he needs to do the same thing for you." The two officers referred to the importance of the strong bonds they maintained with their colleagues on the street, mentioning that "we were and we are together ... they were present whenever we needed them…." Furthermore, police officers, who worked on the street with Evans and Victor, showed their respect and recognition for their sacrifice in the line of duty. The two officers stated that their colleagues regularly visited them in the hospital, and that they congratulated them in a genuine way that gave them encouragement to cope in the aftermath of their trauma ("....they really meant that ... they made you feel good...."). Even though emotional expression is not always acceptable by the traditional police culture, it seems that in such moments some officers expressed their emotions openly. They commented,

> "People who worked on the street, really, they were able to understand our situation ... the first day in the hospital a person came ... who was at the same precinct, but he was working on a different shift, we didn't know him in person and ... he was hugging us and ... you were looking at him and he was crying ... we didn't know them, but because they had gone through similar situations they were able to understand.... You see people at the end of their career ... who are still on the street ... and they get touched ... and we didn't know them ... seriously ... I believe that an officer who works on the street and risks her/his life knows what danger means in police work .... and could not remain emotionally untouched by such an incident....."

Discussion - Outcomes

The aim of this paper was to explore the way trauma in the line of duty and re-traumatization during court proceedings were experienced by two police officers. We hypothesized that repeated exposure to trauma would have a negative impact on two officers' mental and physical health. We identified potential protective factors that helped the two officers cope with the aftermath of the multiple trauma experience.

Protective Factors

The two officers received support from their family members, friends, and others, who were genuinely willing to show them empathy. They also received recognition and encouragement from their own colleagues, who were able to identify, to a certain extent, with their experiences. The solidarity and cohesiveness of the police culture enables officers, even the most experienced ones, to express their emotions. The two officers were acknowledged by their colleagues for their bravery since they risked their lives to maintain peace and order. The support coming from their friends, family and colleagues, was especially significant for Evans and Victor to recover and cope with their traumatic experiences.

The path from the edge of death to the "psychological fire" of the trial was characterized by support from others on one hand, and by isolation, on the other hand. Therefore, they return to the "second round" (the trial), just the two of them, ready to confront the "psychological fire" as they did with the real fire while on duty. It is these moments that manifest the strong bonds of trust and love of their partnership that helped them cope with the trauma and re-traumatization. The unity and ethic of care from one partner to the other is also accompanied by self-reliance that gave them strength to support each other as well as their families. Another protective factor of importance was the fact that the officers felt physically well after their hospitalization. Physical recovery helped the two officers to feel better psychologically as well, which is an example of the connection between the mental and physical health.

Trauma and Re-Traumatization

Evans and Victor experienced flashbacks, nightmares, sense of "feeling stuck" in the trauma experience, and re-experiencing the event. Their effort to hide their own trauma, is not only related to their symptoms but is also expanded to the re-experiencing of the near-death experience, and the trial. They went to court by themselves, asking their significant others to stay behind, so as to protect them against a situation that would be painful and, perhaps, traumatic. In their effort to appease their close friends and family that things were getting better for them, they tried to pretend that everything was fine ("You need to show them that you are strong. You must not show them that you go through pain. In other words, you need to pretend that you are ok.....").

The case of Evans and Victor challenges the policies and procedures of many police organizations. A superficial interpretation of such a situation is that this is merely part of police work, and things need to "move on." Such a perspective invalidates officers' experiences and may stigmatize their potential efforts to ask for psychological help. Evans and Victor were expected to recover within a certain amount of time after the exposure to adverse incidents. In this case, psychologists of the organization were supportive and open to help the officers and their families, but it seems that their willingness to help was not sufficient to convince the two officers to seek out psychological support, since they only attended a few sessions before dropping out.

In summary, this case demonstrates the need for further research and discussion in the exploration of this unique cumulative form of trauma experienced by the police. This will lead to the development of programs that provide the awareness and validation of the potentially re-traumatization experience associated with being required to testify in court while facing the perpetrator. These programs would enable officers to become more familiar with the role of mental health professionals within the police organization and, vice versa, allow mental health professionals to customize their services to the unique nature of police work and the testifying procedures required of first responders.

REFERENCES

Andersen, J., Wade, M., Possemato, K., & Ouimette, P. (2010). Association between posttraumatic stress disorder and primary care provider – diagnosed disease among Iraq and Afghanistan veterans. *Psychosomatic Medicine, 72,* 498-504.

Hall, G.B., Dollard, M.F., Tuckey, M.R., Winefield, A.H., & Thompson, B.M. (2010). Job demands, work-family conflict, and emotional exhaustion in police officers: A longitutinal test of competing theories. *Journal of Occupational and Organizational Psychology, 83*, 237-250.

Huddleston, L., Stephens, C., & Paton, D. (2007). An evaluation of traumatic and organizational experiences on the psychological health of New Zealand police recruits. *Work, 28*, 199-207.

Kingshott, B.F., Bailey, K., & Wolfe, S.E. (2004). Police culture, ethics and entitlement theory. *Criminal Justice Studies, 17*(2), 187-202.

Komarovskaya, I., Maguen, S., McCaslin, S.E., Metzler, T.J., Madan, A., Brown, A.D., Galatzer-Levy, I.R., Henn-Haase, C., & Marmar, C.R. (2011). The impact of killing and injuring others on mental health symptoms among police officers. *Journal of Psychiatric Research, 45*, 1332-1336.

Orth, U. & Maercker, A. (2004). Do trials of perpetrators retraumatize crime victims? *Journal of Interpersonal Violence, 19*(2), 212-227.

Papazoglou, K. (2013). Conceptualizing police complex spiral trauma and its applications in the police field. *Traumatology, 19,* 196-209.

Rudofossi, D. (2007). *Working with Traumatized Police Officer-Patients. A Clinical's Guide to Complex PTSD Syndromes in Public Safety Professionals*. Amityville, NY: Baywood Publishing Company.

Sugimoto, J.D. & Oltjenbruns, K.A. (2001). The environment of death and its influence on police officers in the United States. *Omega - Journal of Death and Dying, 43*(2), 145-155.

In: Listening to their Voices of Bravery
Editor: Konstantinos Papazoglou ISBN: 978-1-53610-048-8

Chapter 2

POLICE OFFICERS BEING HELD HOSTAGES ON A PEACEKEEPING MISSION: EXPLORING A UNIQUE FORM OF POLICE TRAUMA

Monica Ghabrial [*] ***and Konstantinos Papazoglou*** [†]
University of Toronto, Toronto, ON, Canada

INTRODUCTION

> "I realized that something was happening to me, I couldn't control it. It was like ehh…it was like ehh…an old-fashioned ehh…gramophone…when you walk the same line all the time…"

Police have been deployed internationally for several years for various services; yet, there is little research regarding the effects of peacekeeping work on their physiological and emotional wellbeing. Police peacekeeping work has been considered a form of community policing where communities experience "civil war, communal violence, or the erosion or collapse of effective government…and the police keeping role becomes one of peacebuilding…"

[*] Psychology PhD Candidate in Health and Minority Groups, University of Toronto, Toronto, ON, Canada.
[†] Psychology PhD Candidate in Clinical-Forensic area, Vanier Scholar; Police Captain (former) Police Academy, Hellenic National Police and European Police College.

(Grabosky, 2009, p. 101). Police offer a special set of skills and experiences to UN peacekeeping missions, as they are prepared with very specific training and philosophies. They are qualified to be available, responsive, and fair to the public – working and mingling within the community, and responding promptly and respectfully to appeals of the local population (Bayley, 2011). This unique background contributes to a breadth of available sources for peace support; however, police are not traditionally prepared for military roles and the diversity of national police services can make international interaction and communication difficult (Greener, 2011). Bayley (2011) suggested that the main purpose of the police within the military is not to act as soldiers, but rather to support the local governments by tending to the safety of civilians.

Peacekeeping operations (PKO) workers have a range of responsibilities and potential stressors. Generally, they may fear being unable to adequately help the local population (Britt & Adler, 1999). PKO workers witness death, starvation, illness, and great need, leading to feelings of powerlessness, helplessness, and anger. They may also vicariously experience feelings shared among the local population, such as rage and despair, resulting in secondary traumatic stress disorder (Wessells, 1998 as cited in Shigumera & Nomura, 2002). As peacekeepers, these police are also instructed to use no force, except for in self-defense. Though they may be subjected to shootings, hostage situations, and other hostile encounters, they are unarmed, and must restrain their reactions. Distress may then result from this need to be passive and restrained in the face of life threatening and unpredictable situations (Dirkzwager, Bramsen, & Van Der Ploeg, 2005).

Despite the fact that PKO workers operate under such stressful and volatile conditions, related health issues are rarely addressed and seldom researched. Research that has examined mental health issues in military psychiatry, has found many accounts of posttraumatic stress disorder (PTSD) and war neurosis (commonly referred to as "shell shock"; Shigemura & Nomura, 2002). Peacekeeper's stress syndrome is also formally acknowledged as a unique problem of UN peacekeeping, and is defined as, "rage, delusion, and frustration, feelings of impotence and helplessness when confronted with violence and atrocities to which the peacekeeper is unable to respond." (Pearn, 2000, p. 435) A variety of other psychiatric diagnoses or specific psychological conditions have also been reported; for example, acute stress disorder, PTSD, conversion reaction, posttraumatic depression, alcoholism and drug abuse, somatization disorder, lifestyle and cultural change syndrome, chronic peacekeeper's syndrome, and survivor's guilt syndrome (Pearn, 2000). Because demands on police and PKO workers are so high, they are at great risk for mental health issues; yet, it is because of their high-stress roles as peacekeepers that they must be of sound health and mind.

Police and military cultures heavily influence experiences with combat zones and peacekeeping, as well as the recovery process following traumatic events. Both cultures foster stigma surrounding mental health issues and services, which often means that these resources are not fully available and that many individuals avoid seeking much needed consultation (Sharp et al., 2015). Masculinity has long been considered a critical principle of military culture and individuals are discouraged from discussing work matters in an emotional context. It has been suggested that these masculine ideologies have great impact on the suicidal behavior found in the military (Braswell & Kushner, 2012).

Summary of Cases

Steven. At the time of the interview session (January 2014), Steven was 57 years old, married, and had two daughters and two grandchildren. Steven and his family lived in a Nordic country. By the time of the interview, he had worked with his home country police for 33 years. Steven (pseudonym) was stationed as a UN police protection force in a self-made Serbian republic located in Croatia during the Balkan War. On the evening of May 24th, 1995, Steven began back home after a full day on duty. Steven was staying in private accommodations at the time and, as part of a UN protection force, was unarmed. As he and his colleague sat on the balcony of their home that night, discussing the events of the day, they observed as four Serbian guerillas in camouflage approached their residence and stood before and discussed the UN vehicle parked in front of Steven's residential building. Suddenly, one of these unknown guerillas ran into a neighbor's home and began an argument, the topic of which Steven could not discern. Following this man's return to the group, the four Serbian guerillas charged at the UN residence, kicked down the door, and entered in combat formation. Steven detected that something was wrong and instinctively threw his wallet with his money and passport under the bed. The Serbian guerillas reached the second floor, where Steven and his colleague had been, and pointed their Kalashnikov rifles at them, ordering them to the floor. The Serbian guerillas then took Steven and his partner's uniforms, which would presumably be used for night raids of Croatian areas. In only their underclothes, Steven and his colleague were taken, at gunpoint, to the UN vehicle. Steven was ordered to drive to Devoir – an area nearby his residence - and the group of them drove, as the intoxicated gunmen drank and sang war songs. He was eventually ordered to stop in an area known for landmines. Steven and his colleague were then forced out of the car and ordered to walk into this area. As the two stood there unclothed in the dark and cold, the Serbian guerillas announced that they blamed the UN for supporting the Croats and that they would kill Steven and his colleague to make a statement about this perceived injustice. The four guerillas then fired their rifles into the air above Steven and his colleague and drove off in the UN vehicle, laughing and leaving the unarmed and unclothed Steven and his partner standing among the landmines in the dark. The two officers found their way safely back to the road and wandered in the night until they came upon a controlled area with UN soldiers.

Nelson. Nelson (pseudonym), our second interviewee, was 61 years old at the time of his interview and had been working as a police officer for 38 years. He was married, had four children, was also residing in a city located in a Nordic country, and was working as a police officer. In January of 1995, Nelson was deployed as a UN peacekeeping officer to east Slovenia – a village central to the zone of separation – during the Balkan war. On March 18th of that year, Nelson received an order to drive with a colleague to UN headquarters, about 50 kilometers north of where they were stationed, to retrieve a newly deployed officer. Next, Nelson and his two colleagues set off to the Russian military camp; however, before they reached their destination, they came across a parked car, which was blocking the narrow road. Their jeep approached the unidentified car, unable to pass due to ditches on either side. The people with this car then suddenly surrounded the UN jeep, shouting at the three officers, tearing open the doors, and taking their belongings and weapons. Nelson told us that one of these men grabbed him and held a pistol to his head. Nelson and his colleagues were then ordered at gunpoint to drive until they reached an abandoned barn. The three UN officers were pushed inside and told that they must not leave the decrepit barn for one hour, lest they be shot by snipers waiting outside. Their abductors left the house, locking the officers inside. Nelson reported that he and his colleagues immediately rushed to escape the house, somehow managing to unlock the doors. As they suspected, they found no one waiting outside, and began their journey towards the Russian military camp on foot. When they reached the camp, they came upon an Irish engineer who was eating lunch, but were reprimanded for disrupting his meal and told to wait.

FINDINGS

There were eight themes that arose during the two interviews, which were divided into three sections: 1) Unique nature of police work in peacekeeping missions, 2) Experience of trauma in police culture, and 3) The aftermath of trauma.

The Unique Nature of Police Work in Peacekeeping Missions

Both interviewees discussed the unique nature of peacekeeping mission work. Often, the unpredictability of this work was addressed as something idiosyncratic to warzones. As a result, peacekeeping soldiers must have strong and reliable instincts; they must be prepared for the unexpected and alert to unusual or potentially threatening changes in their surroundings. For example, when the group of disguised soldiers approached his residence, Steven detected that there was a threat: "They made in combat formation, into our house, and up the stairs. And I said to my colleague, 'Oh, oh…something is very, very wrong."

We examined Steven and Nelson's interviews for similar experiences and sensations. Both interviewees experienced a sudden lack or loss of control early on and both were held at gunpoint. Nelson described how a routine procedure turned swiftly into a life-threatening event:

> "And we went through very flat open countryside and I-I-I-I been there quite many times so it was just routine to go out there. And we didn't expect any problems. But then, in front of me, I saw a car uh strangely park across the-the narrow road, ditches on both sides. So [I] went up there, and the next thing that happened was the people up there, they was surround our car with-with masks on and started shouting, opening-tearing off the doors and uh weapons out front. And I recalled that one he grabbed-took hold of me and I had a pistol up here to my head…"

Both Steven and Nelson also experienced a distortion in their perceptions of time and surroundings, which included memory gaps and loss of time. For example, "Then suddenly they have masks on they-they prepared for this--It was very--Everything was very fast," and "I could recognize the face but from where, at that time, I didn't know. After…I don't know, 15 minutes? Half an hour? I don't know."

During the incident, Nelson noted that he felt two things: concern for his teammates and anger towards his abductors. Throughout the abduction, he remained conscious of the whereabouts of his colleagues who were with them, and showed concern for their wellbeing. Nelson thought always of his fellow soldier: "And then short after we're looking at each other I guess we're all relieved that they did not shoot us, and I-I was mostly thinking of the newcomer…[stuttering] separation for him."

In Steven's case, his captors subjected him and his colleague to humiliation, in addition to threats. Their uniforms were taken and they were forced, at gunpoint, to stand in a minefield.

> "And I was in underwear and so was my colleague. And they ordered us to go down to the river and I knew that if I did that I will walk into a minefield. And we stepped out and when we were standing there they started to laugh at us. And one of them said to us 'Yeah, you are happy. You can go home. We live in this warzone, we can do nothing. We have our families, we have no food, we have no medicine, we have nothing to our families."

His captors felt that they were justified in their actions because of the injustices that they had experienced and the conditions that had become a part of everyday life. Steven added, "And then they started to talk about the…uhhh…the unfortunate war for them and the… that the UN police were helping the Croats and now they had to create an example by killing us."

Although warzones are stressful and unpredictable, there appears to be desensitization to the horrors that can occur. This can lead to a lack of sympathy and support in the community. When Nelson and his colleagues sought help after being released from captive, they met with soldiers who were unfazed.

> "So we continued and reached the-the-the Russian camp in the outskirts. We got in contact inside it was like uh…I … got in contact with somebody having lunch, or whatever it was, and they turned out to be Irish engineers. They ask us not to interrupt their lunch, come back later, I thought that we were being [punked]…come back little later…"

The desire for closure was a notable remark made by Steven. Although he and his colleague were told by their captors that they would be killed, they were not, leaving him to question the reason for the torment they had been put through. He asked, "But why give us that experience, why do that to us?"

Experience of Trauma in Police Culture

Police culture is often dominated by macho values; that is, trauma experience and related trauma symptoms may be accepted with skepticism by other police officers. Steven appeared to be hesitant in sharing his traumatic experiences with his colleagues because "police officers are very [emotionally] closed people…they don't show feelings." Thereby, his need to speak up was precluded by his fear of being humiliated by his own colleagues: "So I think it's quite normal. I think every colleague, eh… in the beginning, I was thinking if don't… If I tell them about it, will they look at me in another way? Will they say, 'Oh he's a pussy.' " On the other hand, Nelson was confronted with denial when he escaped from his hostage place to seek out safe shelter into a Russian military base:

> "…we continued and reached, the-the-the Russian camp in the outskirts we got in contact inside it was like I…I… got in contact with somebody having lunch or whatever it was and they turned out to be Irish engineers they ask us not to interrupt their lunch, come back later"

It also seems that Nelson did not receive any special support in his own military base because what happened to him and his colleague was considered routine, or another incident among so many that had happened before: "They carried on with the work…It was another incident…Nothing special." Yet, bureaucratic processes following the incident seemed to be in high priority "…[I was] brought back to the Headquarters in order to report what had taken place…and being interviewed by the military police…and it took all afternoon, all evening." Back at the military base, Steven's colleagues took steps to ensure that he was physically well and provided him with necessary materials (e.g., blankets) as well as basic (or rather superficial) emotional support:

> "And we came in and they were, 'Ahhhh, what they do to you?' And they gave us blankets and they were made report to the headquarters, the

military headquarters…and a peach – a preacher. And, uhh… they took us back to our old base. Our old base, where we were stationed also. And they tried to talk with us and tried to give us a little…'Now it's over, you are safe now, and nothing is going to happen now.' "

Once again, Steven's experience was not considered a work-related incident, but rather a regular incident expected to happen: "…My incident was not reported as a work-related incident…" Further, the day after his traumatic experience, Steven was ordered to work the nightshift "at a police station, remote… and I was standing along…sitting along…there was nobody else…" Although Steven received very little emotional support at his military base, some of his colleagues were able to show understanding. Steven explained how this surpassed his expectations, "…Will they say, 'Oh, he's a pussy?' No, no. Nobody ever did that. Ever. Nobody even…I don't think anybody even thought that. I think they have accepted that I have been on the edge." Unlike Steven, Nelson did not receive this kind of support from his colleagues. In contrast, he felt stigmatized by some of their comments: "Yes, it was– It hurt me more than I actually realized. After my…I spoke with colleagues, they said – yeah – they could see I started to look different…They could see something was wrong." In addition, he reported using alcohol on the first night of his traumatic experience: "The same day [of the incident] in the evening…everything ended up in alcohol."

Feelings of shame and pride motivated both Steven and Nelson to participate in a new peacekeeping mission after they returned home from their traumatic peacekeeping mission. As Steven stated, "…Inside my head, I know I have to finish what I started." This common narrative suggests that the drive to successfully complete a mission is a part of police identity. Nelson mentioned that, "I was ashamed with that ending with my mission…" and Steven emphasized his own police pride and perseverance that he had to complete the job: "It is a pride…you know, you are very…as a policeman you are very…I am a little special (chuckles)…If I say I do it, I do it." Indeed, Steven referred to his wife's words when he made the decision to return back to the warzone: "Steven, if you don't go back, you will blame yourself the rest of your life that you didn't finish…You cannot live without doing and finishing what you have started." Following his wife's encouragement to complete the mission, Steven concluded: "I would have blamed myself that I didn't go back. So I went back."

After the completion of his peacekeeping missions, Steven became a peer-support coordinator in his area. He argued that police culture has recently seen a shift from the traditional macho values it once held. He explained, "Nowadays, they don't ask you [if you need to talk to somebody] they tell you that you have to talk with somebody...I think they [the organization] are much better now than they were before." Steven contended that police officers should feel comfortable speaking with a mental health professional about traumatic experiences; he mentioned that talking to a mental health professional about trauma should be considered a normal procedure because police officers are "normal" human beings: "You have to realize that life is like a glass…Your soul is like a glass. Every time you have an experience – bad or good – the water is dripping." He continued, making this suggestion to his peers:

> "I want them [other officers] to learn the lesson that no matter what you are, you are not more than [a regular human being]…things can go wrong. Don't believe that because you are a police officer, that you are made of a special kind of…ingredients."

In similar lines, Nelson's message to other police officers who have been exposed to trauma was the following:

> "…be aware of it [trauma], it can show up, be very careful about how you maintain your daily work…Be aware of how you feel…and don't neglect it…I thought it was–nothing would…would knock me down but it really did…It can happen to you. No matter how you think about yourself it may hit you."

Trauma Symptoms

Both Nelson and Steven reported multiple symptoms related to their traumatic experiences in the warzone. Steven referred to incidents that triggered his traumatic memories; specifically, he noted a time when his police colleagues disguised themselves with military attire and set off fireworks for a surprise celebration to welcome him home: "…I was crying and I was thinking about [the incident]…and I didn't tell them that I was crying – but they thought it was tears of joy." In the line of duty as a police officer in his home country, Steven mentioned that certain moments would have triggered him to overreact with civilians "…I could feel that when I was in special situations during…night shifts…If I came out and there was something…a perpetrator with a gun…I could overreact in a way…"

Uncontrollable emotional expression (especially crying), intrusive thinking, and physiological reactivity relevant to the incident seemed to have been some of the main trauma-related symptoms described by our interviewees. Steven described his "unharnessed" periods of crying without having been able to identify the reason behind his tears: "I was crying all the time…and for no reason my world started to pshhhhh…everything, I was crying for nothing." Steven also referred to his post-war visit in the place where he served as a peacekeeping officer. The place itself triggered traumatic memories and, in turn, he experienced physiological reactions: "I was sweating like a pig, because I thought all kinds of things would happen." Further, Nelson mentioned that after he return to his home country, he was compulsively preoccupied with listening to the radio for news on the peacekeeping forces: "I had the radio going on all the time listening for news…a lot of news from Bosnia…and finally my wife said, 'I am throwing that radio out…Stop it, let it go, you are back home now.' Even when I went on the bathroom I brought the radio up there to get the latest news…I couldn't let it go."

Steven recalled the time when he felt numb, avoided everyday tasks, and was easily irritated:

> "…I was not participating in anything…I was lying down, I couldn't eat, I couldn't sleep, I couldn't…and I could lie on the couch, looking in the air for hours…my wife said 'Hey, what about the lawn…?' 'Maybe tomorrow, maybe tomorrow…' But this [trauma] wouldn't go away. I felt that when the children was doing something wrong, I was very (snaps fingers) quickly to be angry."

Both Nelson and Steven struggled with nightmares and insomnia for years after their exposure to trauma. Nelson reported his insomnia experiences vividly: "I was really sick from not sleeping and I found it difficult to sleep. I woke up, fell asleep, woke up so many times during the night…I hated the look of my bed; that became kind of my enemy (laughter)." Consequently, Nelson was unable to concentrate in his workplace and often felt fatigued: "I…I um got more and more tired…"

Almost 20 years have passed after Nelson and Steven were exposed to their traumatic incidents and, to them, it seems that recovery is a life-long process: "It was a long, long, long journey…and I am still travelling and…I am still travelling...today."

The Aftermath of Trauma

We asked Steven and Nelson about their coping mechanisms and the long-term effects that their traumatic experiences had on their lives. Steven described the change in his perspective of police work back home following the incident; no threat seemed quite so sinister in comparison to his peacekeeping experiences and he had a new appreciation of life. He explained:

> "And I would say to myself, 'Calm down, it is nothing. Nobody is killed, nobody has been shot or something like that.' And I felt that… I could feel that something happened to me, that I was back in… when something like that happened, I was thinking, 'But down there, they were killed… they disappear – people…but here, nothing happening.' And appreciate that I live in a country where … we have a democracy…and a stable society."

He also found comfort in a higher power and explained that, because he had survived so many life-threatening situations, he felt as though God was protecting him. Writing and journaling was listed as a comforting exercise, which helped Steven remember and come to terms with the details of the incident. He added, "Writing is my therapy…" Both Nelson and Steven used the services of a healthcare professional following their traumatic experiences. Steven, urged by his wife, sought the help of a psychiatrist, who normalized his symptoms and prescribed medications for his Post-Traumatic Stress Disorder (PTSD). Being able to discuss his problems with a professional, he said, has enabled him to speak openly about the event without feeling his PTSD symptoms – which included physical pain and temporary insomnia. He described the effectiveness of his treatment:

> "What was important for me was that he said to me, 'Steven, it's quite normal. What you have… the experiences that you have had…the way you react – nothing unnormal [sic] in that. It's quite normal to react in the way that you did.' Just to hear him tell me, that the way you react is normal."

Unlike Steven, Nelson did not feel a significant benefit from seeing a mental health professional and did not pursue this form of treatment. Instead, he consulted a medical doctor regarding insomnia. His doctor also normalized his symptoms, and prescribed medication for his sleep disorder. With the encouragement of his psychiatrist, Steven continued to find comfort in sharing his experience with his family, friends, and colleagues. He discussed his strong feelings about open communication and the effect that talking about his experience had on his health and growth, as well as the consequences he feels can occur if one chooses to refrain from discussing one's trauma:

> "I think… the fools who have a negative result, it's who doesn't talk about it and try to eh…to press it down. And I think if I didn't talk about it and I didn't do-did something about it, I think I would have…I don't think I would be in the police force today. Because I think if…if I would have let the experience take control, I don't know where I would have ended. I took control and I am still here."

Recreational and leisure time was mentioned as an important coping mechanism for the symptoms of both interviewees. Compartmentalization was critical for Nelson, and he focused on maintaining a separation of work and home life. He listed karaoke, kayaking, cycling, and fitness training as therapeutic activities. He also told us that he and his colleagues drank a considerable amount of alcohol on the evening of their incident. He said, "We talked about it like police officers do," and that they drank in such excess that "everything disappeared." Steven found comfort in time spent with his grandson, as well as recreational activities with his colleagues. He also dedicated time to his community. When he returned from his peacekeeping mission, he started a youth support group and eventually became Head of Education for police cadets in his area. Another way that Steven worked to cope with the trauma from his event was by revisiting and taking vacations in Croatia. "I think I'm stuck with Croatia," he said. "It's like [my] country." Steven described the climate and landscape of the area with fondness, and went on to say that he also collects pictures from the region where he was based.

Acceptance was another common theme between Nelson and Steven. Both interviewees accepted that such events were common hazards of peacekeeping work regardless of training and preparation. Further, these incidents have had lasting effects on them that cannot be fully undone. Steven said:

> "I will tell you about some incidents that I have had, which made me realize that no matter how well-prepared you are, how well-trained you are, you cannot avoid getting in situations that you can't control…It will never go away, it will always be a…It would be a part of my life, but I've learned to live with it."

Steven told us that he felt guilt for leaving his family and placing them in a situation in which they may have been left fatherless. "I wanted to have this experience," he said. "I was thinking more about myself than I was thinking about my family." However, in addition to acceptance, Steven showed forgiveness – for himself and his captors.

> "I don't blame myself and I don't blame the Serbian guys anymore. In the beginning, they were the bad guys. Oh, I tell you, I was wishing a lot of things for them. But now, I'm…I feel a little sorry for them, that they have come to me in the situation, that they have to do so– things like that to a human being."

Steven also told us that this experience gave his family a new perspective of police work, changing how they perceive coping and trauma. "And I think she [his wife] also realized that, [just] because you are in the police force, that it doesn't mean that you handle everything." Both interviewees also highlighted the benefits of maintaining a positive environment as part of their recovery. Nelson described his determination to keep in good spirits and to have this reflected back to him by others, as well as the fulfillment he receives from contributing to his community and training other officers, internationally. Steven mentioned that his emotions are reflections of those around him and, thus, he always works to improve the wellbeing of others. One way that Steven became more invested in the wellbeing of those around him was an increased protectiveness of his daughters. This desire to create a positive environment is also what motivated him to participate in research and programs that aspire to improve conditions and treatment for officers who have had similar traumatic experiences. However, Steven also found difficulty in the lack of true understanding he received from those around him.

> "When you tell anybody else about it, they will say, 'That was a hard one.' But they will never be close to understanding what it really means. 'We're glad that you didn't get killed'…But I don't think that they can understand it."

When asked what advice he would offer to others in his line of work, Nelson suggested that other officers take the time to be mindful, present in the here and now, and to observe their surroundings:

> "Try to, um…to evaluate this situation – you know, what is going on. To calm down a little bit…and to look and listen and observe what is going on. And…then normally-normally, somehow, when I'm in a new strange situation something usually shows up in order to get through this situation in a good way to solve the problem."

DISCUSSION – CONCLUSION

Police work is generally challenging and police officers are often exposed to potentially traumatic incidents in the line of duty. Police officers are deployed as peacekeeping officers in violent and politically hostile contexts; hence, they often experience numerous adversities. As Steven noted, such adversities - or else potentially traumatic incidents - are often unavoidable and unpredictable when an officer is deployed in a warzone or, otherwise, areas of conflict. Our interviewees indicated that traumatic incidents are treated by the peacekeeping organizations as "normal or expected or usual incidents." That being said, Nelson was taken to the local UN Headquarters to report the incident to the military police and Steven was provided with blankets and clothes and then he met with a religious preacher who tried to provide support. They were cynically told that the incident was something normal that would possibly happen while on duty; they just needed to finalize the bureaucratic processes reporting the facts, and it was checked and confirmed that they were physically well. As a result, both interviewees were treated by their organizations in a way that further isolated them and forced them to suppress their emotional pain. Specifically, the day following their traumatic events, Steven had to work a nightshift alone in a remote police station and Nelson consumed alcohol to alleviate his emotional pain. Nevertheless, regardless of rank and professional experience, traumatic incidents such as those experienced by Nelson and Steven are not everyday job hazards. Indeed, our interviewees stated that their traumatic experiences were unprecedented and had malicious effects on their personal – as well as their professional – lives. As aforementioned, Nelson and Steven experienced multiple trauma-related symptoms that affected their lives for many years following trauma exposure occurred.

Despite their suffering, Nelson and Steven felt obligated to remain silent and perform their duties out of pride; that is, they had to prove that, as police officers, they were not psychologically affected by "normal and expected incidents" during a peacekeeping mission. After they returned to their countries, Nelson and Steven chose to reapply for deployment on new peacekeeping missions. What motivated them was their obligation, as officers, to complete their mission successfully and eliminate any residual feelings of shame they may have felt from their previous mission.

Nelson and Steven managed to cope with their trauma symptoms in a constructive way. For instance, they positively re-framed their relationships with their families, they developed healthy social networks with friends and colleagues, and they sought help from healthcare professionals. In addition, Steven displayed altruistic social advocacy, helping youth in his community to get involved in sports and other social activities. He also became police peer-support program coordinator in his hometown.

What could be improved? The voices of Nelson and Steven led us to a few possible clinical and policy recommendations for police officers deployed as peacekeeping officers. Peer-support programs could be developed during peacekeeping missions. Through these programs, peacekeeping officers exposed to any traumatic incidents may have trusted colleagues with whom they can share work- and trauma-related stories and stressors. Moreover, it is imperative that on-going psychological support is available during peacekeeping missions, not only to officers exposed to traumatic incidents, but also to any other officer who wishes to benefit from the services of a mental health professional. Regular psychological assessment would also aid in examining the potential need for psychological support. Likewise, rigorous psychological training before and after deployment to a peacekeeping mission would highlight the importance of psychological self-care, as well as possible techniques that would help them improve their resiliency and promote their health; hence, they will be able to prevent the blatant impact of extreme stress and trauma on their wellbeing and job performance.

References

Andersen, J. P., and Papazoglou, K. (2014). Friends under fire: Cross-cultural relationships and trauma exposure among police officers. *Traumatology*, 20(3), 182-190.

Bayley, D. H. (2011). The morphing of peacekeeping: Competing approaches to public safety. *International Peacekeeping*, 18(1), 52-63.

Braswell, H., and Kushner, H.I. (2012). Suicide, social integration, and masculinity in the US military. *Social Science and Medicine*, 74(4), 530-536.

Britt, T. W. and Adler, A. B. (1999). Stress and health during medical humanitarian assistance missions. *Military Medicine*, 164, 275-279.

Dirkzwager, A. J. E., Bramsen, I., and Van Der Ploeg, H. M. (2005). Factors associated with posttraumatic stress among peacekeeping soldiers. *Anxiety, Stress and Coping*, 18(1), 37-51.

Grabosky, P. (2009). Police as international peacekeepers. *Policing and Society*, 19(2), 101-105.

Greener, B. K. (2011). The rise of policing in peace operations. *International Peacekeeping*, 18(2), 183-195.

Pearn, J. (2000). Traumatic stress disorders: A classification with implications for prevention and management. *Military Medicine*, 165(6), 434-440.

Sharp, M., Fear, N. T., Rona, R. J., Wessely, S., Greenberg, N., Jones, N., and Goodwin, L. (2015). Stigma as a barrier to seeking health care among military personnel with mental health problems. *Epidemiologic Reviews*, 37, 144-162.

Shigemura, J., and Nomura, S. (2002). Mental health issues of peacekeeping workers. *Psychiatry and Clinical Neurosciences*, 56(5), 483-491.

Wessells, M. G. (1998). Humanitarian intervention, psychosocial assistance, and peacekeeping (pp. 131-152). In: H.J. Langholtz (ed.), *The Psychology of Peacekeeping*. Westport, CT: Praeger Publishers.

Woody, R. H. (2005). The Police Culture: Research Implications for Psychological Services. *Professional Psychology: Research and Practice*, 36(5), 525-529.

In: Listening to their Voices of Bravery
Editor: Konstantinos Papazoglou
ISBN: 978-1-53610-048-8

Chapter 3

ONCE "BLUE" ALWAYS "BLUE": A LAW ENFORCEMENT PROFESSIONAL THWARTS MASS SHOOTING IN A PUBLIC PLACE

***Raquel Hudson*[1], *Marian Pitel*[2,*] *and Konstantinos Papazoglou*[1,†]**
[1]University of Toronto, Toronto, ON, Canada
[2]University of Guelph, Guelph, ON, Canada

INTRODUCTION

> "I'm just now, six years later from the shooting, starting to emerge from the cave I've been hiding in."

Who do heroes call when they need to be served and protected? The answer for most heroes, is no one. Law enforcement officers face a wide range of critical incidents over their careers (Kingshott, Bailey, & Wolfe, 2004). These incidents often vary in type, oscillating unpredictably from short-lived, acute situations to more complex, multifaceted events. Of the more complex critical incidents, the mass shooting is of particular interest to first responders, public/social media as well as the public in general due to its premeditated

---

* Master's candidate in Industrial-Organizational Psychology.
† Psychology PhD Candidate in Clinical-Forensic area, Vanier Scholar; Police Captain (former) Police Academy, Hellenic National Police and European Police College.

nature and the high volume of victims and witnesses typically involved. These critical incidents may debilitate and isolate individuals who experience it due to its unique nature.

Due to the extremely stressful nature of these events, it is not uncommon for survivors of mass violence to experience trauma-related symptoms. Bardeen, Kumpula, and Orcutt (2013) reported that intense post-traumatic reactions are felt in the acute aftermath. Law enforcement officers, however, are chronically exposed to traumatic events, causing an accumulation of symptoms and trauma exposure instead of dissipation. How the symptoms affect officers through their everyday life is significantly based on a dynamic exchange among perspective about the traumatic experience, resilience, and the desire for change.

Scientific literature has examined how individuals are affected psychologically by mass shootings; however, the sample population has been limited to civilian survivors (Fox & DeLateur, 2013; Norris, 2007). In a similar fashion, post-trauma resilience and coping of police officers and other first responders have been studied in a general police patrol context (Pole, Kulkarni, Bernstein, & Kaufmann, 2006); nonetheless, little is known about the unique experiences of former and current officers surviving a mass shooting incident. In this chapter we will uncover the voice of a hero, who had to face a mass shooter alone in her – open to the public - workplace.

Rachel's Story

> "Even though it's tough to talk about some of this stuff, I'm doing it cause I know you're going to help people and you're going to make it so that cops don't have to suffer like I did."

Rachel (pseudonym) was the sixth born, into a large family with seven siblings. She grew up in a highly educated and affluent family. Despite Rachel's family being established and large, Rachel felt unloved. She felt different from the rest of her siblings and she knew she was. Subsequently, as a child, Rachel would comfort and befriend the outcasts, because she wanted to ensure that everyone was happy. Adversely, Rachel would be systematically sexually abused from the age of four until young adulthood through molestation and rape. As an adult, Rachel would come to identify as a lesbian and never been married.

After trying out several programs in college, Rachel graduated with a bachelor's of arts in criminal justice with a minor in psychology. Shortly after,

Rachel answered her calling to be a law enforcement officer. Rachel moved up quickly in her department, however, her ambition was faced with contention.

Rachel faced various episodes of depression and "darkness," but chose to see the "light" at the end of the "tunnel." As a strong believer in Jesus Christ, Rachel was assured that she did not have to face life's challenges alone.

Rachel was an adventure-seeking, confident, brave yet still humble woman, who decided to face death, due to her innate call to duty and service. Now in her mid-40s, Rachel's life would be drastically altered. On a cold Sunday morning Rachel's destiny aligned with purpose and she was able to overcome the gunman and save thousands through - what she referred to as – "divine intervention."

Rachel had been off duty the day of the incident, when her intuition and unconscious cues from prior experiences, awakened her and drew her into work where thousands of people had access publicly. Rachel served as a sworn law enforcement officer for more than a decade in major US metropolitan cities. Despite being the only officer to defend thousands of civilians against the gunman, Rachel remained poised and focused.

When she arrived at her workplace, the gunman had already begun to shoot civilians. While gathering information from surrounding witnesses, Rachel was alerted to the presence of smoke outside of the building's front doors. Moments later, the loud echo of a high-powered rifle (an AR-15) filled the air. Rachel pulled out her gun from the waist band of her jeans and sprinted towards the gunman.

The hallways of the building were chaotic, people were screaming, people were frantically trying to hide and run away from the gunman. Yet, Rachel described those moments, as "the hallway being empty, silent and just the gunman, God, and her." In the midst of chaos Rachel was able to focus and calculate each step towards the gunman.

Finally, Rachel confronted the gunman, with confidence that she had come prepared and was not going to die. Rachel and the gunman exchanged gunfire, after the gunman refused to back down. Through calculated steps, the shooting ended when Rachel's bullets fatally wounded the gunman. From that moment on, Rachel would become the hero that saved thousands from not only the gunman but several explosive devices planted by him - around Rachel's workplace premises - before he started shooting the crowd.

EXPLORATION

The Survivor's View of the Adverse Incident

Facing Death

Rachel faced death and conquered it through positive self-talk as she confronted the gunman. Rachel told herself during the incident "I'm not going to die. I'm going to kill this guy, he's not going to kill me…I'm not gonna die, he's going to die." Despite Rachel being the only police officer on the scene, she remained confident while facing the gunman by reassuring herself that she would defeat the gunman and knowing that God was with her. That was all she needed. Furthermore, Rachel's strong spiritual connection to God led her to believe that she did not have to face death alone. Rachel said during the incident "I asked God to be with me…God is the reason I didn't get shot. The gunman shot at me several times, but missed. I know that is because God protected me."

The Aftermath

Rachel stated that she had trauma-related symptoms following the incident. Firecrackers on holidays sounded like gunshots. When people surrounded her to thank her for her courage, instead of engaging in conversation with them Rachel mentioned that "I could not hear them and not because I was losing my hearing, but because I could not focus. I was somewhere else in my mind. This lasted for several weeks. I had no idea what was happening to me." She withdrew socially and even stopped going to church. Rachel also experienced trouble with sleeping, and she recalled not being able to sleep for a long time "I would close my eyes but I couldn't sleep…forever, it took forever." Rachel also described how she felt isolated and abandoned, she stated, "I was totally abandoned…It's very real…I've got post-traumatic stress disorder. And it's not pleasant… I'm just now, six years later from the shooting, starting to emerge from the cave I've been hiding in". According to Rachel, "three days after the shooting, the lies [from the media and police organization] began." She expanded on this by saying that "what traumatized [her] the most was all the lies." Some media outlets referred to Rachel as a security guard and "that grieves [her] deeply because [she is] a police officer…always have been and always will be." Moreover, Rachel mentioned that, despite having faced a number of different critical incidents over her career, "to have [the facts of an adverse event] lied about is the most traumatic thing that could happen to anybody." The aftermath of the mass shooting incident is inundated with an internal dialogue in Rachel's mind about survival and death or life decision that she had to make during the incident:

> "Having to violently end a person's life, though I am a police officer and had no choice, is a very unnatural thing to do. Killing someone has forever changed my life. Yes, I know I did what I had to do and would be able to do it again if needed, but when you're not a murderer and are a person with a soul, it is definitely a most unpleasant experience."

Police Identity

Ethic of Care

The law enforcement mantra is to maintain peace and order. Rachel embodied this mantra, she stated "a privilege and honor to take care of people in the most dangerous situations." Rachel also believed that "I'm responsible as a cop to save other lives…their lives are in my hands." The strong-held belief that she was responsible for others' lives was helpful in providing Rachel with the courage that she needed to defeat the gunman.

Multiple Roles

Law enforcement officers often occupy multiple roles. They typically cycle rapidly among roles; from being crime-fighting conquerors, "social workers," administrative clerks, friends, family members, and romantic partners. The challenge of managing these roles is amplified when they are chronically exposed to threat, which builds psychosocial walls against relationships outside of law enforcement (Patterson, 2003). Rachel stated that "I do isolate myself and I, I don't know if that's a good or bad thing…I just kept it all to myself." Law enforcement officers are trained to devote equal amount of energy towards capturing suspects and preserving their lives. Unless warranted to do so by extreme circumstances, police officers are taught not to compromise their promise to protect all lives in order to apprehend a criminal. As Rachel expressed, "the very person that tried to kill you, you have to save their life after you've shot them… that is the training of a cop."

Thrill-Seeking and Preparedness

Another aspect of the police identity that helped Rachel during the critical incident is familiarity with thrill and adventure. As expressed by Rachel, as a law enforcement officer "I like the dangerous stuff because I know what to do and I do it well. The more stressful the situation the more at home I am because I am in my element." Furthermore, preparedness is essential for officers to possess in order to successfully overcome a critical incident. As Rachel says, "[she is] not afraid to take on another gunman… Somebody tries to kill [her], they're in for a surprise." Rachel also stated that police lifestyle is not for everybody "it's not for everybody, not just anyone can do this job."

Coping Mechanisms

Positive Thinking

Rachel used positive thinking to gain the courage and confidence to confront the shooter on the day of the shooting. Additionally, positive thinking is a general strategy that allowed Rachel to get through life, in spite of the hurdles she has faced in the past. Rachel was "positive and hopeful that God has something really good for [her]."

Reprocessing Thoughts and Emotions about the Mass-Shooting Incident

Rachel was also able to cope by actively reprocessing her thoughts and emotions. What this entailed was Rachel tracing back and recovering the thoughts and feelings that she had when the event happened and then reframing them in a way that is conducive to enhancing psychological health. For instance, Rachel mentioned, "it was so quiet… It was quiet other than the gunman… It was very fast, [she] was calm, not shaking…" Whether or not it truly was quiet at the time, remembering the event in this manner changes one's experience of the incident and removes the negative emotions (e.g., threat, chaos) that were initially associated with the event.

Resilience and Strengths

Rachel remained resilient in the face of adverse events through her faith, optimism, and desire to get better.

God and Spirituality

Rachel's faith in God played an essential role in her daily life and during critical incidents while on duty. According to her, God is "top priority." She believed that it was a part of God's plan for her to be at the [place] that day to stop the shooter from killing any more civilians. Furthermore, she argued that "God is the reason [she] didn't get shot." With "His help," she was able to stay calm during the incident and maintain focus on stopping the mass shooter. She went on to also mention that without God, she definitely would have taken her own life. Given the number of times so many people and so many in the media have betrayed and lied about her and this incident, doing their very best to discredit her not only as a person, but as a police officer. Given the number of negative experiences Rachel has had in the past, these words indicate the protection and security that she attributes to God and her religious faith.

Hope

Rachel recognized the importance of being optimistic despite the challenges that one had to face. Rachel stated that "you can say poor me or you can say no, I've got a lot to offer this world… I do have hope, otherwise I'd be dead." Her hope was also as strong as her faith, Rachel expressed that "hope will keep me going."

Self-Reliance during Recovery

Another strength of hers that is as unwavering as her faith and optimism, is her intrinsic desire to recover. When asked about motivations to recover, some people turn to extrinsic reasons like seeking treatment for the well-being of one's children or being compelled by one's partner to speak to a counselor. In contrast, Rachel expresses that she's "getting healed because [she believes in herself and wants] to get well."

Sharing and Recognition

Empowerment through Recognition

Rachel stated that some media outlets and police officials masked her bravery by providing skewed reports of what happened during the incident. However, not all of the post-event reactions were negative from a psychosocial aspect. A few days after the mass shooting, Rachel was formally praised by city officials and received multiple standing ovations. Of all the positive responses she received from different individuals, the most salient was the invitation that she received by the US President's office to be honored by the President himself for her bravery during the mass shooting incident. As stated by Rachel, "there was an amazing presence in the midst of us when I got to meet the President and he said, 'Good job, I'm proud of you.' " According to her, "it meant a lot because he didn't listen to all the lies." Additionally, law enforcement officers from across the globe continue to reach out to her via social media and email so as to thank her for her heroism during the mass shooting incident.

Value of Sharing Her Story

The value that she places in sharing her story to the world is unparalleled. Rachel stated:

> "Even though it's tough to talk about some of this stuff, I'm doing it 'because I know you're [refers to the chapter authors] going to help people. You're going to make it so that cops don't have to suffer like I did, and other cops did."

Whether it's through her writing, interviews, or other projects, Rachel has worked hard to ensure that other officers can take something away from her experiences that will benefit them if they ever have to face similar situations.

DISCUSSION – RECOMMENDATIONS – FURTHER ACTIONS

Despite experiencing trauma-related symptoms following the incident, Rachel was able to persevere through resilience, which protected her from severe negative health outcomes. As part of her strong law enforcement identity, Rachel's ethic of care kept her driven to save lives and her mental and physical preparedness allowed her to remain calm and focused, in spite of the life-threatening situation that she faced. Coping strategies such as survival thinking (in Rachel's case survival thinking was manifested as positive-hopeful thinking) and situational reprocessing of thoughts and emotions about the incident also aided in buffering the negative effects of her trauma exposure. Rachel's strengths, including, among many, her spirituality, her unconditional hope, and self-reliance for recovery, served as protective factors and helped her remain resilient. Consequently, her past experiences of injustice and victimization conditioned her to feel empowered through adequate recognition and find value in sharing her experiences with others.

Aside from sharing her personal story, Rachel was also keen on identifying critical issues within police organizations, specific to trauma exposure and treatment. The first issue that she identified was the need for more post-traumatic stress disorder (PTSD) prevention and treatment programs for police officers. As Rachel expressed, "there's no prevention or resilience programs for cops." She argued that unlike police officers, soldiers and veterans have been offered disproportionally more PTSD therapy programs compared to police officers, who experience a unique form of complex trauma. Rachel argued that:

> "Police officers are typically in very close proximity to the perpetrator when they are forced to engage and kill. Soldiers are typically much further away. Soldiers don't have to see the eyes of the person they are about to kill like police officers do. Believe me, this definitely has an impact on the officer. Forever."

Secondly, she expressed the need for specialized training for psychologists who work or aim to work with police officers. Specifically, Rachel stated:

> "I've seen a lot of death by gunshots and... [The bullet] shreds your face or your chest or your arms or your legs. And that is shocking to see...But when we see it all the time, it's not shocking anymore. But...the psychologist is not going to know, they're not going to have a clue. No matter how descriptive you are, they're not going to get it... You would traumatize the therapist if they watched [videos of real death] but it's almost like you have to see the most graphic, violent deaths in order to understand what the cop or the soldier had to do... otherwise, they're not going to have a clue."

This last passage from Rachel's interview highlights the need for psychologists and other health care professionals to receive specialized and sensitive training that can compensate for the lack of visceral exposure to the type of events that police officers and other first responders regularly face. Rachel concludes her interview with the following words that she needs "to be heard" through the lines of the present chapter:

> "I have never had anyone-ever-to talk to about the shooting. Not siblings, not friends. This has been devastating. That, along with how much my incident was so completely distorted by many in the media and others, has traumatized me further. This has caused my continued

isolation-especially when certain things trigger me. All of this has also delayed my healing. What I don't understand is why people won't allow me to talk about it. It's almost as if they're ashamed of me. At least that's how they've made me feel. I simply did my job as a well-trained police officer. I didn't ask for anything in return. Especially not to be betrayed by so many."

CONCLUSION

Rachel's case emphasized the necessity for further research in examining the unique form of chronic trauma experienced by law enforcement officers. It highlighted the importance of cultivating in current police officers the factors that protected Rachel from extreme and prolonged distress in the aftermath of her traumatic experience. Rachel's story also demonstrated the mind-body connection between positive cognitive thoughts and external overt behavior, through her use of positive self-talk to maintain control during the mass shooting incident as well as other challenges in her life. Future resilience training programs with emphasis on special care about police are necessary to provide law enforcement officers with adequate support.

REFERENCES

Bardeen, J. R., Kumpula, M. J., and Orcutt, H. K. (2013). Emotion regulation difficulties as a prospective predictor of posttraumatic stress symptoms following a mass shooting. *Journal of Anxiety Disorders*, 27(2), 188-196.

Fox, J. A., and DeLateur, M. J. (2013). Mass shootings in America: moving beyond Newtown. *Homicide Studies*, 20(10), 1-21.

Kingshott, B. F., Bailey, K., and Wolfe, S. E. (2004). Police culture, ethics and entitlement theory. *Criminal Justice Studies*, 17(2), 187-202.

Norris, F. H. (2007). *Impact of mass shootings on survivors, families, and communities*. National Center for PTSD.

Patterson, G. T. (2003). Examining the effects of coping and social support on work and life stress among police officers. *Journal of Criminal Justice*, 31 (3), 215-226.

Pole, N., Kulkarni, M., Bernstein, A., and Kaufmann, G. (2006). Resilience in retired police officers. *Traumatology*, 12(3), 207-216.

In: Listening to their Voices of Bravery
Editor: Konstantinos Papazoglou

ISBN: 978-1-53610-048-8

Chapter 4

EXPLORING THE EXPERIENCES OF POLICE OFFICERS WHO DEADLY SHOT SUSPECTS IN THE LINE OF DUTY

***Negin Sohbati*[1,*], *Monica Ghabrial*[2,†], *Konstantinos Papazoglou*[2,≠] *and Peter Tam*[3,‡]**
[1]University of Toronto - Ontario Institute for Studies in Education (OISE), ON, Canada
[2]University of Toronto, ON, Canada
[3]John Jay College of Criminal Justice and Hunter College of the City, University of New York, NY, US

INTRODUCTION

"I had been asked to make a split second decision, suddenly everybody else was gonna be determine what my life was gonna be for the rest of my life." Ted.

---

* Masters of Teaching candidate.
† Psychology PhD Candidate in Health and Minority Groups.
≠ Psychology PhD Candidate in Clinical-Forensic area, Vanier Scholar; Police Captain (former) Police Academy, Hellenic National Police and European Police College.
‡ Adjunct Professor, John Jay College of Criminal Justice and Hunter College of the City, University of New York, NY, US; Police Sergeant – Office of the Commanding Officer – Police Academy New York Police Department (NYPD).

"I didn't do this with hate in my heart and I know that I guess that's what allows me to keep going, you know. I wouldn't be able to carry the thought of taking a life…." Tony.

Over the course of their careers, most police officers find themselves making critical decisions under extreme stress in the line of duty (Anderson, Litzenberger, & Plecas, 2002; Broomé, 2013). "Shoot or don't shoot?" incidents are one example of such critical situations in which a life or death decision must be made. It has been found that police officers can experience extreme levels of anxiety when faced with an armed and uncooperative suspect (Anderson, Litzenberger, & Plecas, 2002). Officers are mandated to assess every encounter and use situational information and evidence to formulate a course for action (van den Heuvel, Alison, Power, 2014). This means that officers are authorized to use lethal force when it is legally justifiable to do so (Broomé, 2013). "Shoot or don't shoot?" incidents often lead to extreme stress, which can be detrimental to an officer's clarity of thinking and subsequent decision making (Nieuwenhuys, Savelsburgh & Oudejans, 2012). Many officers who have been involved in deadly force shooting incidents reported changes in their thinking, behavior, and perception in the aftermath of such incidens (Artwohl, 2002; Honig & Roland, 1998; Honig & Sultan, 2004).

SUMMARY OF CASES PRESENTED

Ted. In the late 80s, a 34 year-old police officer's life changed dramatically. At the time, Ted (pseudonym) served at a major metropolitan police service in Western Canada and he was married with two young children.

The incident began when Ted received a call reporting an armed robbery at a bar. Ted and his then partner located and followed the suspects' vehicle. Once with the alleged robbers, Ted decided to call the local dispatcher in order to confirm the suspects' descriptions. Upon overhearing the dispatcher's voice over Ted's radio, the suspects fled the scene. Left with no other choice, Ted and his partner engaged in a high-speed chase until the suspects' vehicle crashed into three parked cars. In an attempt to flee on foot, one of the two suspects got out of the car and attempted to flee. Despite Ted's clear and direct commands to stop running and surrender, the suspect continued to run. The suspect eventually jumped into parked car with his hands concealed in the front of his jeans. When the alleged robber made a move toward Ted's partner, Ted made the instinctive decision to pull the trigger in an effort to protect his partner from whom he thought was an armed criminal. He fired a single shot at the suspect, dropping him to the ground immediately.

After the shooting, Ted remembered hearing the other offender surrender as other officers began to arrive on scene. After searching the deceased suspect thoroughly, Ted realized that there was no gun to be found. Seconds later, Ted was informed by his supervisor who had just arrived that he was under criminal investigation for manslaughter.

Tony. In early 2012, Tony (pseudonym), a 32 year-old police officer, who served in a major US Northeastern metropolitan city for almost five years, received important information that would transform what was originally a drug surveillance operation into a firearms arrest. Tony and his team followed a suspect into his apartment where a series of adverse events unfolded. Despite being held at gunpoint, the suspect refused to withdraw his hands from under his shirt, where Tony believed he was hiding a gun. After much resistance, and despite Tony's many demands not to move, the suspect sidestepped into an adjacent room, which was outside of Tony's field of vision. Not knowing what the presumably armed suspect was doing in the other room, and with only a layer of drywall between them, Tony made the instinctive decision to pull the trigger before the suspect had a chance to act.

It was later found that the suspect had been unarmed and the District Attorney decided that this case would be treated as criminal and that the routine legal proceedings would follow.

FINDINGS

Immediately After the Shooting: Organizational and Legal Procedures

Both Ted and Tony were expressly critical of the rigorous organizational and legal procedures that they had withstood immediately after the shooting. They reported being stripped of their firearms and escorted back to the station where they were asked to report the details of the shooting. They both vehemently conveyed their frustrations about this, claiming that it had been extremely difficult for them to concentrate and gather their thoughts on paper just minutes after the shooting. Both officers described feeling restless as they racked their brains for the details of what had happened. Right after the incident, both Ted and Tony reported that they felt unsupported by the organization as well as a number of their own colleagues. For both Ted and Tony, investigations followed the incidents. Tony: "…enough time had passed where the ambulances were there. There's about 150 cops outside already…. It was a chaotic scene….and the platoon commander takes my firearm…" In Tony's case, the union representative asked him to "shut up and sit down in the car," because anything he would say might be used against him during the investigations. Nonetheless, Tony argued that he was ready to undertake the responsibility of his actions. He said, "I did the most severe thing you could do to another person and….I want to be held accountable if I was wrong. I want to be accountable." Tony reported that he felt more agitated because authorities were withholding information on the condition of the suspect he shot: "Nobody wants to give you a straight answer … Why won't you tell me? On the other hand, Ted described with disappointment: "I found out that my suspect was declared dead by hearing the Staff Sergeant and Inspector arguing between the two of them which one of them was going to tell me. Turns out they didn't have to tell me since I heard their argument [about my case]…" In similar ways, Tony described: "… and, I actually found out, I was in the hospital and I just happened to see the news on the TV." Similar to Tony, Ted described the paradoxical situation that he experienced right after the incident: "Lots of profuse sweating and perspiration and worry about everything… The union association says, 'Don't write anything,' and the lawyer comes in and says, 'Don't write anything,' and then the police inspector comes in and says, 'Give us a report…don't say anything, but then tell us everything.' And what a hell do I do?"

Tony described his absolute frustration about being taken to a psychologist with whom he was to speak about the incident and his mental and emotional state, despite being warned that nothing he divulged to the doctor would be kept confidential. Tony's frustrations are best captured in this statement, "The police department brings you in and sits you in front of, you know, a psychologist and tells you that anything you tell them is not confidential. And you're so afraid, between the court side, you know the actual legal side… and the department side." Similarly, Ted noted: "I was offered absolutely nothing by way of psychological assistance. I wasn't even asked if I needed such help …" Ted and Tony both expressed their utter disappointment about what they considered less than sympathetic treatment from their organizations. They explained that the organizations seemed to be more concerned about the logistics of the event, rather than the mental and emotional state of their colleagues and employees.

Symptoms in the Aftermath of Trauma

In their interviews, Ted and Tony both revealed that symptoms of trauma plagued their everyday lives, hindering their recovery. One of the most salient symptoms they both described was insomnia and subsequent restlessness. To explain this, Ted said, "It felt like I would fall asleep in exhaustion for about five minutes. Then, I would wake up in a panic and I would pace back and forth for hours until my legs were exhausted again physically and then I would fall back asleep and wake up five minutes later and it would start all over again and it was like that all the time."

Another symptom that both officers endured after the incident was hypervigilance. Tony described feeling very threatened that he might be assaulted or attacked whenever he was outside of his house. To give us a better understanding, he gave this example: "I got in my jeep and started driving …. and this guy's driving, like, right behind me flashing his high-beams and I was just enraged, I felt in a very threatened. Like, 'I'm mad because I feel like you're gonna hurt me' … And it was just …. typical city driver." Further, Tony mentioned that he became fixated with monitoring the verbal and body language of people around him when he was in public spaces. Hypervigilance often caused him to avoid crowds by staying at home, rather than spending time with his girlfriend in public and social settings. Nonetheless, his hypervigilance was aggravated by the fact that some individuals recognized him in public and assaulted him verbally. He provided examples of things that these people might say to him: "…I know who you are. You are the cop that shot that kid. You are going to jail. They're going to fire you in like two weeks." Ted claimed that he was always prepared to deal with the worst case scenario when he was on duty saying, "For my whole career on the street after that, every time I turned a corner, I was ready for a bank robbery. I knew where every bank was, where every gas station was, where every pharmacy was in my area – so every time I turned a corner, I was ready for that split-second decision that had to be made."

Another symptom that both Ted and Tony described during their interviews was time distortion. They both explained that a major struggle when reporting the details of the event was placing the events in chronological order. To describe this, Tony said, "I mean, if you go into the tape … the time frames are all weird. I've had a hard time figuring out dates and months; it might all be jumbled and confusing." Toward the end of his interview, Ted made a stunning revelation. He disclosed that despite all the support he had received during his recovery period, there were days where he felt extremely overwhelmed and anxious; this drove him to contemplate suicide. Ted went as far as planning to kill himself on a day when his wife and kids were out. Fortunately, his wife, who noticed that Ted looked depressed and extremely stressed, suspected that Ted required immediate attention; she called a colleague and close friend of Ted's while she was at work and asked him to visit Ted at home. That day, Ted was quite literally saved by the bell as his friend arrived just before he was about to commit suicide:

> "I remember deciding that I was thinking the best thing I could do is to commit suicide and so I had prepared for that.... So, I went to the basement to plan out my suicide and .... I had great sense of relief.... it was this great sense of relief of I finally figured out this is gonna work well for me ... so I went down to the basement to revisit the whole plan to make sure I thought things through and the doorbell rang and I ignored it, (knocks) door pounding ... pounding ... pounding, 'Ted, open the door.' It was [Ted's colleague]. He had been an officer-involved shooting who had talked to me several times and was a friend of mine.... I finally came out of the basement and answered the door and he said, 'What are you doing?' and I said, 'I can't ... I can't keep going, that's enough.' And he said, 'Stop, stop talking like that, that's not right.' And we sat down and we chatted and we chatted for several hours, I think. And finally, my wife came home and I was okay ..."

Nature of Police Work

> "I had no idea how heavy the uniform was until I finally took it off for the very last time due to retirement, knowing I would never have to put it on again....When I slept, I think I almost slept for about three months when retired..." – Ted.

A general experience of police work is the instability and unpredictability of any given – especially critical - moment. On-duty officers can spend several hours of a shift, doing mundane and routine patrolling in the neighborhoods. While most or all of a shift can be uneventful, when the time comes to take a call and work a case, things can quickly progress to a highly chaotic state. To communicate this, Ted shared with us a common saying in the force: "90% boredom; 10% full bore chaos." Considering the amount of shifts an officer works throughout his/her career, this can result in multiple complex traumas. Our interviewee, Ted, compared this to the experiences of a civilian:

> "In normal life, most people will have 2 or 3 traumatic things happen to them for the whole life…In policing, there's 200-500 traumatic events that can occur in your career … So I have 300 events that can trigger me now. The thing is, is that, at what point am I strong enough to be able to recover from the trigger and still work with it?"

Police officers often work in challenging contexts in which they must make acute observations in their environment and quick and effective decisions about the necessary actions to take. Tony explained to us that he was stationed in a neighborhood in which residents avoided cooperating or speaking with police; thus, making cases difficult. This makes observing and studying the environment especially critical to making decisions in this context. Furthermore, an action that proved effective in one context might be damaging in another and officers cannot generalize and apply the same methods to each situation. Tony described:

> "You watch people as they move, as a cop, and everything is an observation…my biggest fear was that guys would see … I didn't hesitate and the guy didn't have a gun, and I'm in the position I'm in ... that doesn't mean the next guy won't have a gun."

Our interviewees also discussed the tendency for officers to idealize their work. Tony told us that he was deeply invested in his work because he had previously encountered civilians who reported feeling unsafe in his district because of dangerous and questionable elements in the neighborhood. He said that his mission became to "hunt" those who posed a threat to the safety of the area. He said:

> "I felt like that was actually the real police work that you read about and you see in the movies and it's like, 'This is what I'm doing. I'm doing the actual police work.' I mean, you answer complaints… loud noise; boyfriend, girlfriend beating each other up … But this is like the crux of what and I enjoy – I loved it."

Two themes that appeared in association with the idealization of police work were an "Us versus Them" mentality and the rationalization of violence. Tony mentioned that officers also tend to rationalize violence using the "Us versus Them" mentality. "I have good friends. I've one good friend who's like, 'There's a lot of people who are—'like, a lot of my friends are military, cops … you know … They're like, 'He deserved it …''' Officers also appear to use the idealization of police work to rationalize this violence, feeling as though fatal incidents and casualties are the cost of protecting the peace. Tony reported: "I mean, some people making jokes, as sick as it sounds, like, 'He's a perp .... he's a perp ...' I'm like, 'Dude. Doesn't matter if he's a perp ...'"

In spite of this idealization of police work, officers can find themselves disheartened by the lack of support that they receive from the force. Tony told us that in many cases, an officer might feel as though the police force punishes them for self-defense or minor mistakes. As an example, Tony told us a story of a female officer who shot and killed an unstable perpetrator who was assaulting her with a chair, and was subsequently penalized by her department. Tony also explained that officers are punished for minor errors made on duty that, otherwise, have no negative impact on the case at hand. Specifically, Tony noted: "But if... if everything else was good, why are you looking for something bad? Why are you looking specifically to hurt the cop?"

This shift in treatment and perception was also addressed by both participants in terms of being labeled as either a "hero" or a "zero" in the police force; however, Tony and Ted each had a unique view and experience with this dynamic. Tony explained to us that one is considered a "hero" when tasks and cases are being performed perfectly and without fail; yet, when an officer faces an obstacle and falters or takes an action that causes negative consequences and bad press, that officer is then treated as a "zero." In terms of the "hero" or "zero" dichotomy, Tony mentioned:

> "I got my pick of assignments 'cause, you know, I was an active guy. It's like when you're giving them what they want, you know, when you're giving them the arrest numbers ... you're an active cop, they love you. Until something goes wrong ... You feel like you're being punished. Again, it's one of those things where you're treated like a ... like a number. You're treated like a pariah ... You know, it's like ... I'm literally just a file on a desk."

Ted, on the other hand, told us that he and his colleagues changed the stigma and dynamic by reclaiming these terms in a support group comprised of those who might typically be considered "heroes" and those who would not. Ted reported:

> "So ... we got together, the seven of us. Some us had been shot and survived and some us had shot other people. So, we called ourselves the 'heroes and zeroes.' You were a 'hero' because you got shot and

everybody felt sorry for you or you were a 'zero' 'cause you shot somebody and you were investigated for a criminal offense … But what we realized is that whether you were a 'hero' or a 'zero' when we talked to each other, we felt the same; we felt abandoned, we felt misunderstood, we felt that we had to put on a façade of being well when we knew we were not well … There were no resources available to us ..."

One source of stress that Ted revealed to us was the tendency in police work to be wholly absorbed by police identity and "live blue." He explained that those who fully subscribed to the lifestyle, in which officers must consume themselves with their work, are completely disconnected from any personal life. According to Ted:

> "Blue is the complete disconnect from the community and just associating with people who are working with you. Police officers, they become your family, they become your friends, they become the only people you can talk to, they become the only people you will work with, the only people you will have fun with … and so what happens is, you live, eat, breathe, a trauma- induced life 24/7, 365 and how long can the brain take that?"

A prolonged and extreme exposure to violence compounded by the lack of external community, support, and outside interests and enjoyment, often renders officers susceptible to burnout and isolation. To explain this, Ted shared a story about a young officer he once knew who he believed had suffered these consequences. While on duty, this officer chased a suspect into a river, and the suspect subsequently was drowned. The officer, while under investigation and accused of racism towards the deceased perpetrator, found himself with no support or protective factors. Ted shared his perspective of this case:

> "He was so blue and so proud of policing that he put them on such a high pedestal…that when that happened to him, he felt he had shamed the uniform. And that was one of the things kept eating at him and eating at him, 'cause he kept saying to me, 'I've shamed the police. I'm so sorry. I shamed the police.' And at some point he said he wanted to go rock climbing with a friend of his and he went home and shot himself ... I attribute his wanting to give up to being blue and not being able to disconnect from being blue."

Because of stories like this, Ted now uses his position on the force to ward officers away from this "living blue" mentality. Ted prepares new recruits by first alerting them to the great responsibility they are being given and ensuring that they are aware that this work does not benefit them with special rights or privileges. Secondly, Ted reminds the recruits that they were hired based on character and their individual traits and histories, and to not lose sight of this during their careers. He added:

> "The second thing I would say to them: 'You joined the police service because we like you and I'll tell you what we liked about you: we like your upbringing, we like your contacts in the community, we like your volunteer work, we like your social work, we like your education, we like your participation in sports, we like your family structure. If you throw all of that away to become a police officer and can only hang around with police officers now because now [you're] just a police officer, that's a breach of contract, because we didn't hire you to be blue –we hired you for everything you bring to the organization …'"

However, although the tendency to "live blue" is common, Ted noted that police culture has been shifting away from emphasis on this mentality. As new generations of recruits who are older and educated enter the force, there is a decrease in complete assimilation and blind loyalty.

Specifically, Ted explained:

> "Why there's a bit of a revolt now is because now we have people who are old enough to say, 'Well, hold on a second here. I am 27 years old, I've been doing some studying, I've already got my family, I've already got my financial portfolio, I've already got some things in place. I'm not sure I'm gonna be blue.' So, there's a bit of a revolt now of people who are saying, 'No, you don't own me. I just work for you and I only work for as long as I'm happy …' So, there's a change happening now; this thing about blue is going to deteriorate now. Unless, unless they become very aggressive in preaching the philosophy of, 'you can only trust another police officer.' Well, I don't believe that, I don't believe it ever since my shooting. I think there are some very good people in the community who care for you as an individual and they need to be part of your life."

Decision-Making

Another major theme that emerged from both interviewees was the process of *decision-making* they experienced during their event. Both officers addressed their training and the critical role that these procedures played in their actions. Tony said, "Now at the time of the shooting, I reacted the way I was trained. So, training is very important, I truly believe that we need to train police officers for muscle memory." According to both of these officers, the experience was highly physical, from the first alert over the radio to events immediately preceding the case. Tony told us that his body reacted to the call and that this is a common experience:

> "You know, heart starts pumpin', adrenaline starts pumpin', 'cause we know we're going into a –Now, it's a… it's not a typical drug sale like we're used to going after. It's someone with a gun, which is… raises the stakes a little bit." He told us that, during the chase, this physiological response continued. "I was tense… I know I was sweatin'. And I know it was instant, 'cause we weren't physically—You know, I ran ten feet to the door, that was the only real physical thing I did." Ted also illustrated the noticeable tension and perspiration during and directly after the incident.

In addition to these physiological reactions, Ted and Tony shared with us their emotional and psychological experiences. Tony discussed the sense of threat and vulnerability he felt during his event, as well as the experience of facing death. He described, in detail, the many repetitive thoughts he had while waiting for the perpetrator to take action from the other room.

"I'm sittin' here, thinkin' to myself, 'I'm gonna get shot.' It felt like it's fifty-fifty. I felt, at this point, no longer does the police have the advantage. The body armor didn't matter, the firearm didn't matter. I'm at a fifty-fifty. And my thing now is, if I can't see him, I don't know what he's doing. People aren't typically aggressive to people with guns unless they have guns." He told us that he spent these moments wishing for the case to be over, focusing on his finger resting on the trigger of his gun, and thinking of how his family would go on if he were killed on that mission.

> "I pictured it all in my head: Dinner table, Thanksgiving, Christmas time … me not there. The family's there; dogs are running around and I wasn't there. I pictured my girlfriend walking my dogs without me, you know ..."

Ted and Tony both also reported experiencing dissociation, manifested as memory gaps, tunnel vision, and time distortion. During the department's review of his case, Tony was informed of many actions he took and things he said during the event, of which he claims to have no memory. For example, "Apparently, and I found this out later, that I yelled 'gun' right before I shot …" In addition to this, Tony was unable to recall jumping over a baby carriage while chasing the perpetrator, and could not recall distinct details of the perpetrator's apartment. Both interviewees reported experiencing tunnel vision during the event. Tony said, "There was almost no connection with my body. My body, I think, was —The best way I could describe it was, like, I was looking through, like, a camera, like a video. It was like my body was just acting autonomously." Tony also reported time distortion, saying that at times the experience felt as though it were lasting "forever", and that, "…some periods of time in there felt an instant and some periods of time in there felt like they were half an hour to an hour long."

Similarly, during his interview, Ted told us that he felt himself suddenly dissociate just as he was taking action:

> "I didn't even hear the shot go off and then the shot happened retroactively. So, I'm thinking, 'When did I hear it?' And then, when I turned, when [the shift commander] touched my shoulders to say, 'I'll take over from here,' I looked up at him and I wondered, 'How the hell did you get here? Where'd you come from? How long have I been here?'…. I looked up to see police officers running around the scene getting things done, police cars with roof lights flashing, there was an ambulance there and a fire truck …'When did they all arrive?' I didn't see them arrive, I didn't hear them …" About the immediate period following his event, he said, "The next hour was very disconnected from reality. Sometimes I couldn't hear what people were saying … I was [having] tunnel vision."

Ted illustrated his distorted perception of his surroundings during the incident:

> "So, I got all this happening at once and there's this big tree in my way between me and the bad guy and the tree is in my way ... I went back a week later [after the incident] to look at that tree. That thing wasn't even an inch in diameter and I thought this huge tree was in the way – so, just to show how perception is so out of whack. I also wanna share with you, when I shot my gun, there was a lot of smoke that came out, but no sound and then THEN all of a sudden it was like a canon – holy shit! You know?"

Tony also reported this prolonged dissociation after the shooting had taken place. "I walked out, everything was almost muted at that point. I don't know if my ears were ringing a little bit, but it was almost that sensation like, you know, you hear a loud sound like a gunshot without earplugs in, um … just like a very, uh, spacey kind of feeling … Sounds are muffled more than usual. And I was just in a fuzz. Like, what energy I had felt nervous ..."

Adapting to the New Reality

Life following Ted's and Tony's traumatic experiences is marked by desperation and isolation. Ted planned and attempted suicide and Tony mentioned that in such moments of desperation "a lot of guys [officers] go through the cracks… eat their guns… kill their wives and kill themselves…. I am sure they felt like they didn't have a safe place to talk." Their feelings of isolation and desperation deteriorated on the grounds that the lawyer insisted on the fact that Ted and Tony were told by lawyers and union representatives to remain silent about their experiences. Nevertheless, Ted and Tony both noted that they needed to talk to somebody and share their experiences, emotions, and thoughts about the traumatic incident. Ted decided to talk to a priest initially, but he was appalled by the priest's lack of understanding and support, who told him, "Oh, well, God behaves in strange ways…" The priest's superficial answer to Ted's issues led to Ted's agitation and disappointment: "What kind of answer is that? So, that's the best you can tell me?! That God works in mysterious ways?!"

Following the incident and during the investigations Tony was placed in a new position where he worked in a garage where they fixed police cars: "The way they treat you is punitive…I didn't rob a bank, I didn't choose to drink and drive, I didn't choose to beat my wife or my girlfriend." Even after the end of the criminal trial, Tony was confronted with numerous organizational issues that needed to be resolved: "You know, the criminal trial is done, but there is a department trial....they look at your duty status....where they're gonna reassign you." The way Tony was treated by the organization also upset his family: "My mother was, like, destroyed by this...She is like, 'Why are they treating you like this?' and I am like, 'It's just how it works. Just let it go.'" On the other hand, Ted preferred to patrol by himself because he was disappointed by the way his colleagues treated him. Simultaneously, he felt agitated, as he was not aware of his case's progress: "I didn't want to go to work anymore 'cause here's what's happening: I'm driving the [patrol] car and every time the frigging computer would beep, I thought that that would be the beep that they're asking me to come to the station to tell me the decision. So, every time I got a call, I would panic." His agitation was combined with uncertainty about his professional future: "I went into the station, I had to put my gun back on and, every time, I would ask myself the same question 'Is this [shooting] gonna happen again? Can you handle it? Are you ready for it?'.... Then one day I got called in and told that I was being taken off the streets for my own good. I was being re-assigned to Court Liaison...Hell, that's where they put the 'retired-at-work' guys and now I am doing that? I was so pissed, I refused to come in to work. Nobody asked me what I thought, they just decided for me..." Meanwhile, at home, Ted's wife tried to convince him to quit entirely, to shield him from the undue stress. Nonetheless, Ted wanted to prove that he was still strong and able to do the job: "My wife wanted me to quit...I said, 'If I quit now, I admit I can't do the job.' So, I didn't quit... There was pressure for me to appear to be healthy at work....Extremely angry some minutes, crying the next minute....yet putting on a façade of, 'I am fine, I can do the job at work.'" Eventually, Ted confronted the authorities in his organization and insisted on being told of their final decision:

> "I was very angry and I said, 'I am not coming to work until you guys tell me what's happening, because I can't work like this anymore'... I get a call from the inspector and he said 'I'll tell you what the decision is'... I got into the station and he [the inspector] holds the letter like this, 'Here is the letter.' And I went to grab it and he said, 'Just read it'."

What is noteworthy, is that both Ted and Tony observed changes in their colleagues attitudes and behaviors (e.g., avoidance); that is, those colleagues – who were presumably blue brothers and sisters, expected to support them in those grave moments – made them feel alienated and stigmatized in the police context. Ted reported:

"I realized that you stand by yourself …You are no longer part of…no matter how tight you are, you stand by yourself…The police family – you know, we're all brothers and sisters – is only as strong as they are healthy. Once one of them is sick, not so much anymore, because nobody wants to sink with the sick guy."

Tony's description of the way he was treated by some of his colleagues is similar to Ted's:

"They make you feel like a bastard child, like, 'You can't hang out with this guy, he's bad news.' You find out who your real friends are…All of a sudden, you get jammed up, and they don't call you. Then, there's the guys that do and sometimes you're surprised about who that is."

The stigmatization and isolation that Ted and Tony experienced in the organization left them both to feel accumulated anger and tension – which then negatively affected their personal relationships. Tony described conflicts with his family: "But what was getting worse was my, um, my tension … I'd be edgy for nothing …I would get mad about things I don't care about ... I found a lot of things, like irritability ..." Similarly, Ted illustrated frequent incidents of conflict and irritation with his wife: "I came home one day and my wife said, 'What would you like for supper?'… And I blew up and I said. 'Why are you asking me what to make? Why do I always have to make decisions?'… It was moment when the decision-making process should not have been asked of me and I yelled at her, 'Last time I made a decision, I killed somebody.' And I felt so bad…." The aggravated anger, irritation, and tension made Ted and Tony feel emotionally overwhelmed and disconnected from their family members. Ted said, "… You see families fall apart because it's easier to be angry with someone you love than with someone you don't love." These conflicts with loved ones led Ted and Tony to defy the instructions of the lawyers and union representatives. Ted and Tony decided to seek help from a clinician to help them salvage their personal relationships. Tony visited a psychiatrist at the Veterans' hospital and talked to his stepfather, a Vietnam veteran, whom he considers to be a wise man. Over the interview session, Ted became emotional when he described a salient moment during his sessions with his therapist: "He [therapist] said, 'Do you love your wife?' I said, 'Very much so.' He said, 'Are you happy with your family life?' I said, 'Very much so.' He [therapist] said, 'I'm gonna give you some exercises. One of the exercises is that every time you feel overwhelmed, I want to sit down with your wife on the couch and wrap your arms around her and say, 'I need you.' Just be quiet and just let her help you'... So, we just hugged each other and that became my medicine. Constant hugging. Constant hugging."

Effective Coping with Trauma

Through these interview sessions with Ted and Tony, we learned the different ways that each interviewee managed to cope effectively with their traumatic experiences. Tony reported that he prefers to pay attention to positive aspect of everyday life events and exercise different techniques that help him sleep better. Further, he decided to go back to college. Ted noted that he loves cooking, gardening, and making people laugh: "I like to cook ... I have a beautiful garden designed to be peaceful and stress free ..." What is also salient in both participants' stories is that they both were able to appreciate each moment and watch people and things around them and view the positive aspect of their lives. Ted illustrated two distinct moments in his life that were turning points for him in coping with his post-trauma issues (for example, dealing with anger and questioning the meaning of life):

> "...It was on about the sixth year, and I remember stopping at the red light and it was a beautiful, sunny day; people walked around with shorts and t-shirts. And I could hear music in the background and I thought, 'When did the sun started shining?' And I realized at that point that ... the only damage that was happening to me was that I was staying angry. I was causing the problem to myself now. I was my own worst enemy."

> "I hung on to a tree one time and I thought to myself, this tree has been here maybe a 100 years and it's looking very well in spite of what anybody else thinks. So, why can I not live in this world, despite anybody thinking so my tree became my favorite buddy, I'd hug the tree and I'd say, 'you ... you are showing me how I should live...'."

CONCLUSION – RECOMMENDATIONS

In this section, we refer to Ted's recommendations for police organizations, officers, and academia relevant to prevention and recovery in traumatic life-threatening situations experienced by police officers. Ted was one of the pioneers in the development of police peer support programs in Canada and his recommendations also covered Tony's suggestions. In the following lines, we list Ted's quotes that concisely illustrate recommendations for future actions that engage all those involved in police trauma prevention, treatment, and resilience promotion:

- "when people tell me 'oh, I do EMDR…tapping, I do breathing, or I have a dog, or I do horse therapy, or I do painting, or I do yoga, which is best?' All of them are good, whatever works for you. The issue is not to judge others based on what you think. I encourage people to find what is right for them, and not to worry about what somebody else thinks about what they need."
- "police officers need to know that they have to keep their personal connections with the community. It's absolutely essential that they have life lines to support them outside their work as police officers."
- "I would like police understand that they should look to their mental health the way they look their dental health…. they should not wait until they have a rotten tooth to fix the tooth, so should they not wait until they have an injury to fix their brain."
- "I truly think that there are some organizations that are quite willing to try and improve things at work. But some of the officers, frankly, don't want to admit or even take the time to understand that they're in an environment where they can be easily traumatized."
- "If you [officer] get damaged and don't get the help you need, then what good are you to the community?"
- "Many police organizations right now are trying to teach their supervisors to look for signs and symptoms of mental health within the workplace, which I think is a wonderful thing – but I think is a weakness that they only go so far as to develop a training for their supervisors… They need to include families…"
- "They [officers' spouses] have to know that the police organization can and will accept a phone call asking for support on behalf of their spouse without fear of losing their job …"
- "If you teach it [psychoeducation of police stress and trauma] to the recruits from the beginning, as a way that they do business and are expected to take care of themselves, the recruits will believe it …"

- "If you [the organization] tell them that this is a safe environment in which to declare that you have a mental injury, you [organization] better not punish people for declaring they have a mental injury …"
- "You [the organization] have to have an anti-stigma campaign…like the elephant in the room …"
- "need to receive from organization's mental health professionals, validation for changing things within the workplace …"
- "Unless the message goes out from the organization's mental health professionals, then the police organization will always think that their anecdotal interpretation of what is going on is more important than what academia can prove to them."

Ted and Tony's stories provide a rare opportunity for the public, police officials, and clinical professionals to understand two important aspects of police work from an officer's perspective. First, the unique and volatile nature of split-second environments inherent in police work, and second, the traumatic aftermath that follows. These salient aspects of police work are seldom portrayed in the media and many people are oblivious to them. These vivid real-life accounts can serve to inform officers, their families, and police organizations on the reality of the long-lasting emotional and psychological damage that can result from police work and the importance of treatment and attention from mental health professionals and police agencies.

REFERENCES

Anderson, G. S., Litzenberger, R., & Plecas, D. (2002). Physical evidence of police officer stress. *Policing: An International Journal of Police Strategies & Management*, *25*(2), 399–420. doi:10.1108/13639510210429437.

Artwohl, A. (2002). Perceptual and memory distortion during officer-involved shootings. *FfBI Law Enforcement Bulletin*, *10*(71), 18–24.

Broome, R. E. (2013). A Phenomenological Psychological Study of the Police Officer's Lived Experience of the Use of Deadly Force. *Journal of Humanistic Psychology*, *54*(2), 158–181.

Honig, A. L., & Roland, J. E. (1998). " Shots Fired; Officer Involved." *International Association of Chiefs of Police*, June Issue.

Honig, A.L. & Sultan, E. (2004). Reactions and resilience under fire: What an officer can expect. *International Assocication of Chiefs of Police*, December Issue.

Nieuwenhuys, A., Savelsbergh, G. J. P., & Oudejans, R. R. D. (2012). Shoot or don't shoot? Why police officers are more inclined to shoot when they are anxious. *Emotion*, *12*(4), 827–833.

Van den Heuvel, C., Alison, L., & Power, N. (2012). Coping with uncertainty: police strategies for resilient decision-making and action implementation. *Cognition, Technology & Work*, *16*(1), 25–45.

In: Listening to their Voices of Bravery
Editor: Konstantinos Papazoglou
ISBN: 978-1-53610-048-8

Chapter 5

EXPLORING SWAT OFFICERS' EXPERIENCES OF TRAUMA AND RESILIENCE

Marian Pitel[1,*] and Konstantinos Papazoglou[2,†]
[1]University of Guelph, ON, Canada
[2]University of Toronto, ON, Canada

INTRODUCTION

In the previous chapters of this book, we delved into a plethora of different narratives, uncovering emerging themes and exploring the nuances of coping and resilience. Much of the stories discussed are ones of general duty police officers and their experiences with trauma and high stress throughout their careers. Some stories were centered on acute incidents while others explored the aftermath thereof. While there is indubitable significance in studying the effects of acute exposure to critical incidents, there is still a great amount to be learned about the impact of cumulative, high frequency exposure to severely aversive incidents. What currently exists in the literature on this topic is centralized on the effects of trauma exposure on civilian survivors (e.g., Yehuda et al., 1995; Briere, Kaltman, & Green, 2008); the complexity of psychological and physical impact of consistent and accumulative exposure to critical incidents among law enforcement officers is largely unexplored.

---

* Master's candidate in Industrial-Organizational Psychology.
† Psychology PhD Candidate in Clinical-Forensic area, Vanier Scholar; Police Captain (former) Police Academy, Hellenic National Police and European Police College.

In this chapter, we deviate slightly from discussing the work of general police officers and enter the realm of a specialized sector of law enforcement work. In the face of extreme and dangerous situations, patrol police officers may realize that they have limited access to the tactical knowledge and equipment required to adequately eliminate the threat emanated from a critical incident. During these cases, special intervention units (so-called SWAT teams) are often called on scene to help combat the potentially life threatening element by utilizing advanced tactical knowledge and sophisticated equipment (Hudson, 1997). The combination of high incident severity and exposure frequency that is unique to SWAT officers renders their work particularly challenging and may place them at greater risk for psychological and physical consequences.

In a qualitative attempt to shine light on this topic, we uncover the narratives of three SWAT officers from a Nordic country and explore the dimensions of their lives that are affected by cumulative, high frequency exposure to trauma.

EXPLORATION

Personal Experiences

The three participating officers were employed in a Nordic country's Rapid Response Police Unit. We are going to use the term SWAT (Special Weapons and Tactics) for the remainder of this chapter, as this term is widely identified across many police organizations in reference to Special Forces police units. These men shared their unique stories with us and outlined the intricacies of these experiences.

Timothy's Story

Timothy (pseudonym) is a current Federal-level senior SWAT team officer, with over ten years of experience. He has encountered critical incident situations ranging from domestic violence situations to mass school shootings. He has been physically wounded several times over his career and shared two instances with us.

In the late 2000s, his unit arrived on scene to a domestic violence situation. In the midst of crossfire between his team and the assailant, he was struck in the face by shrapnel. As he recalled, "I went… I didn't go into unconscious but it was really close… There was some blood in my hands…"

Months and years following the event, Timothy continued to experience psychological distress. At first, Timothy "was feeling...not angry or anything... [I] was happy that [I] survived that case." However, after four years, the perpetrator "got out... And later on [I] heard that he moved here in the same city where [I] was living..." As Timothy shared with us, that "bothered [me] a while" and this incident led Timothy to carry his weapon for a few months after the perpetrator's release to regain a sense of security.

During that same year, another life-changing event took place. A student entered a high school with a semi-automatic pistol and fired openly, resulting in the death of eight individuals and the injury of a dozen others. Timothy noted that witnessing the death of children in a mass school-shooting event shaped his life differently. Timothy shared with us that "that particular case changed [my] vision about humanity..." As is highlighted by these cases, the two critical events have challenged Timothy's belief systems that are centered on safety and security, both on a personal and global level.

Larry's Story

Larry (pseudonym) has occupied a senior SWAT officer role for over three decades. In several cases, he was appointed as a leading commander of the SWAT operations. Of the several critical incidents he has been exposed to over his career, there are a few that are most significant to Larry.

One instance involved him possessing a commander role in an operation to stop a male perpetrator, driving a vehicle with loaded explosives. He stated that being a leader in a high risk operation was "dangerous" since "it was really... not easy to make a decision because there was no good choices, at all... whatever you do, [anything] can happen." The other critical event he shared with us involved a gunman being fatally shot by his comrades. "When my men shot this guy dead, I was prosecuted by the prosecutor in a lower court and also, the second level," Larry expressed.

Both cases involved Larry facing the consequences of being a leader. For instance, the explosives in a vehicle case placed him in a predicament where a decision needed to be made to continue the operation despite other senior officers telling him to withdraw. In addition, the case with the fatally shot gunman led to Larry going through different levels of court to defend his team's decision to fatally shoot the perpetrator. It is clear, then, that the stress felt in critical incidents is amplified when one is in a leadership role, due to the added responsibility during and following the incident.

Jack's Story

Jack (pseudonym) was a former SWAT officer, possessing a senior role in the unit for over two decades. When asked about the number of critical incidents he has been exposed to in the past, this was his chilling but realistic response:

> Jack: Thousands… But I would say, very dangerous incidents? Couple hundreds.
>
> Interviewer: Couple hundreds? Two hundred, maybe?
>
> Jack: More.
>
> Interviewer: More than that?
>
> Jack: Yeah, more. I have experienced enough… I don't need more. I don't need more.

In contrast to the other two officers, Jack has chosen remove focus from the details of critical incidents and their effects and place it more on what can be done to sever the link between stress and health. "I think this is very important that people who is working… very stressful, very critical incidents, they would understand what has happened inside their body and mind, and how they can prepare, how they can improve their skills, and also mental skills," Jack expressed.

Unique Nature of Police Work

Exposure to Critical Incidents

Police work is unique from civilian work because inherent to the industry is exposure to threatening incidents that are high in severity. As Timothy expressed, it is "very stressful to go through those emotions…again and again. The stress level was always higher." The intensity of these situations renders it difficult to compartmentalize thoughts and feelings related to these events. Timothy added "It always affects you." Larry added to this note and iterates that "you are thinking, all the time… The feeling, it follows [you] several years and even… even now." To add to it, not only are critical incidents high in severity, they are high in frequency. With multiple exposures to threatening situations, Timothy expressed that while "you get professionally better; more efficient, more self-confident," it starts to take a toll on you physically and mentally and it is easy to begin questioning, "Is this the right career [for me]?"

It is even more complex when the SWAT officer occupies a senior role. As a senior officer, Jack explained that "whenever bad things happen, [you are] always first to come in and solve the problems." Many times, there is an extra burden that is placed on the senior officers' shoulders. Larry took on the lion's share of the responsibility when his team fatally shot a gunman and went to court to defend his teammates' decision. In addition, it is common for individuals in supervisory roles to feel partially responsible for the wellbeing of his or her officers. Larry explained that "you have to be really, really sensitive because you really don't know which people need help or support. You have to be really flexible and sensitive to find out who needs support."

Social Network

It is a common phenomenon for SWAT units to feel closer together after encountering the same threatening situations. Timothy described it as a form of "baptism" - a milestone in the police world. It is also not uncommon for personal relationships to be affected in some shape or form following exposure to a dangerous situation. At times, it is a positive transformation. Immediately after encountering severely aversive situations, Timothy's relationship with his wife became "a little tighter...maybe better for a while because you discuss more about things." He added that his wife's support was the "biggest thing that got [him] to go forward... And it really did help." However, there may be potential limitations that thwart post-trauma processing in personal relationships. Partially due to the uniqueness of police work and other parts due to the culture of law enforcement officials, it is often difficult for law enforcement officers to wholly confide in loved ones. As Timothy shared:

> "You can't tell everything to family because, you know, they don't understand everything...It's really hard to try to explain [to] them. Even though a few of them are health care professionals, the situations are pretty different. To get others to understand, it's really difficult."

In addition, relationships can also have negative changes. For instance, Timothy's wife experienced psychological symptoms following the critical incidents. She experienced "symptoms like stress or maybe fears that something happens again." Unfortunately, it is possible for these relationship difficulties to be overwhelming enough to cause irreparable damage in relationships. For instance, Jack explained that he divorced his wife "because of work. I was working...all the time. Think about that, when we have planned weekends together...and then my phone is ringing [for work]."

The Aftermath of the Critical Incidents

It is a fallacy to believe that traumatic incidents have impact on people's lives only when they are immersed in the thick of the situation and that this effect is abolished once the dangerous element is removed from the environment. At times, there are mandatory case-related procedures like court trials that are often stress inducing. Furthermore, there are psychological symptoms that commonly manifest themselves following exposure to such atypical occurrences and may persist as unsolicited reminders of the event for years following the incident.

Post-Incident Trials

Critical situations often involve difficult decisions and might also involve court trials. Larry, for instance, described the court experiences as "stressful, because it is, all the time, going [on] inside you even if you are doing something else and working with operations." Jack has admitted to being in court as a witness multiple times and reports asking himself, "Why I'm here again?" every time he was summoned.

Thoughts, Sensations and Feelings

The first few days after experiencing a dangerous situation, Timothy shared that there are changes to your thinking, both in terms of process and content. He said, "first day or first 24 hours was unrealistic…" Timothy expressed that after experiencing an acute stressful incident, "you can't think about happy thoughts anymore after… You feel great hate feelings towards the perpetrator… You get aggravated more easily." Larry added to this by saying, "it's easier to become upset." He shared that after exposure to threatening events, he was "more tense" and that, "still, twenty-four, twenty-one years after those operations, [he is] still getting better and better."

In fact, Timothy continued this point by noting that physical injuries is not what bothered him the most, but rather, "the mental side that [allows you to be] capable of doing the job was most important." Tim explained this sensation with an interesting analogy: "You shoot a duck or a bird…and the feathers explode. You kind of have the same feeling…Like a bird that was just shot at." A potential consequence of experiencing changes in thought content and processes may be some problems with sleep. For instance, Jack expressed that, "If I have some problems… it is always reflected in my quality of sleep. Sometimes I wake up at like 4am thinking…"

Coping and Resilience

Support from Organization

In order to prevent feelings of alienation along the journey to recovery, it is critical for police organizations to provide the right kind of services to their officers. Post-incident debriefing is one of the most popular trauma-related services offered by participants' home country police organizations. According to Larry, the best type of post-incident debriefing consists of officers gathering together and sharing their roles, failings, and achievements, and afterwards, healthcare professionals presenting the possible symptoms the officers are likely to experience and ways to combat them. He added that, from his experience, tactic-centered debriefing "doesn't work at all." Timothy expressed that while debriefing sessions offered by his police organization were "a little" helpful, the most impactful service that his police organization offered was a general 3-day post-trauma seminar held by a healthcare professional. According to Timothy, the part of the seminar that resonated most with him was the emotion-focused experience-sharing component. He shared with us that his involvement at the seminar "was the first time that you really…got through those…feelings and you get rid of those when you maybe didn't even think about that [before]." He added that the seminar "opened my mind or my eyes" to the psychological effects of trauma and stress exposure and that he would have significantly more symptoms now if he hadn't attended the seminar.

Peer Support

Due to the unique nature of police work, it is sometimes difficult for officers to find people with whom they can share their stories, whether it is to seek advice or to simply unload emotional baggage. For this reason, officers are often more comfortable with speaking to their own peers about their problems. "I don't tell much things to people…Sometimes I discuss certain issues with people, [but] mostly with my colleagues," Larry said. He continued by sharing that he no longer discusses deep issues related to his line of work with his family and close friends. Jack, too, believed that "team members are the best support," because their support is not limited to emotional aid but also incorporates instrumental and tactical components.

Personal Ways of Coping

With the complexity of the stressors that SWAT officers regularly encounter, it is not a surprise that Larry, Timothy, and Jack have all expressed feeling psychological distress at some point over their careers. As Larry expressed, "I used to…somehow, I put [my thoughts and feelings] in a closet in a box and close it… The way I'm living could be somehow easy and nicer after opening them." It is common for individuals to be uncertain of precisely how to effectively manage work-related stresses, like Larry's engagement in psychological compartmentalization as a way to distance himself from his issues. However, from years of trial and error, individuals are bound to come across techniques and strategies that they find, to varying degrees, effective in buffering negative stress-related effects.

The common coping strategy that all three officers found valuable is maintaining physical health through exercise[1].

> Interviewer: How do you cope with stress?
>
> Timothy: "Exercise. And, uh… talk. Those are the key elements."
>
> Larry: "It should be… walking, and, walking every day, for example, going swimming, and wandering in forests and something like that."
>
> Jack: "The main point is healthy. That you… keep yourself healthy. I train a lot."

As is apparent in the aforementioned section, prioritizing one's physical health through activity and exercise is a strategy that is valued by the three SWAT officers in coping with work-related and other life stresses. Although not explicitly mentioned by the participants, it is possible that physical exercise is helpful through its cathartic function. Alternatively, it could also be the related increase in physical readiness for critical incidents that the officers appreciate about engaging in regular physical activity.

A second strategy that was found effective by our participants was spending time with friends and family. As Timothy shared, devoting time to his daughter helps him because it forces him to "concentrate [on] something totally different." While Timothy found it valuable to spend time with family as a way to temporarily distract himself from acute stressors, Jack found that being around his immediate family helped keep him grounded on what he needed to prioritize in his life. Jack noted, "I remember one case where… my boy was like one year old… and that we had very… interesting situation… I don't know the case, what was it, but was a lot of blood… very stressful situation, but when I drive back home, was like fifty kilometers where I live at that time. And I… went home… and I… go beside my boy… and I understood

[1] Although the responses were received from individual, one on one interviews, the participants' responses are clustered at this point for demonstration purposes.

that I really need to change my [senior] role." It is clear that the prioritization of quality time with one's close family circle is highly recommended by our participants.

A selection of cognitive coping strategies was also identified in the interviews. For instance, Jack is an advocate for the use of meditation and mindfulness techniques as a way to prevent and recover from the harmful effects of occupational and operational stress.

> Interviewer: You resolve everything, you arrest the bad guy, then the incident ends. How do you go from this high intensity, high energy level to go down, you know, to calm yourself?
>
> Jack: It's very easy. I can do [that] in just a couple minutes… I just sit down and breathe and... be present. I'm thinking about that I'm sitting down, and I'm breathing, and I'm thinking that now I'm here. It's, um, how can I call it? I transform my mind this moment. Now we are here…. I'm not in the situation anymore. Then [my physiological activity] automatically goes down.

According to Jack, it is difficult for officers to relax and distance themselves from the vividness of the critical incidents they encounter because their minds are trapped in the past ("in history"). Engaging in the practice of mindfulness and meditation is one way to leave memories in the past and to reduce the tendency of negative memories to emotionally debilitate officers. It is apparent in the advice that Jack imparts that one way to minimize the deleterious impact of work-related stresses is to learn about the connection between mind and body.

Recommendations

Recommendations for Professionals in Police Organizations

The three SWAT officers also highlighted some recommendations for police organizations. Initially, there was a request for police organizations to take greater responsibility over the wellbeing of their officers. As Larry expressed, his sole message was that, "organizations shouldn't leave officers alone. They have to take care of them." More specifically, Larry advised that organizations have a contact person responsible for "representing [the] officers and… helping and supporting and coordinating the system for them."

There was a demand for more healthcare professionals with specialized training in trauma and resilience. As Timothy iterated, “there wasn’t that kind of expert…available.” He went on to add that the physician he met with “wasn’t the right person…to understand.” Furthermore, even when he had the chance to speak with a psychologist, “their experience was [in] another field. They didn’t understand that much from the post-trauma situation.” In addition, it is important for healthcare professionals working in police organizations to recognize the stigma present in police culture centered on seeking and receiving psychological treatment. According to Larry, “[going to a psychiatrist] in USA [is an] ordinary thing… but in [my home country], not typical for general and especially not for police officers.” Awareness of this stigma and sensitivity to it is required in order to develop intervention programs that are likely to be received well by law enforcement officers and to prevent intimidating officers from mental health profession’s often biased attitudes held by the public.

Recommendations for Police Officers

Some recommendations for other police officers were also noted. For instance, Timothy gave this advice: “Don’t be ashamed to ask, you know, I don’t know… for help. Even though you don’t feel like needing anything… so… it can’t be worse or bad.” Larry then went on to emphasize the need for organizations and officers to care for their colleagues if an aversive incident is witnessed. He shared the need to support one another by attending seminars and other post-trauma programs together. Larry expressed that, “police officers don’t need to go debriefing in all cases. I understand in some cases, if you don’t need it, and you were close… the operation, it is, sometimes it is important you go there even you are… not willing. Because then you are supporting other people.” He also stated:

> “[In] General, I teach that when… your colleague has been hurt or even killed, or when somebody has been killed, and, for example, shot by police officer. And you are dealing with those officers or their colleagues, or friends, or relatives, uh… sometimes you have a feeling that they behave strangely or even bad. But you have to give them space. Don’t say that they are behaving bad, because there is a million of reasons why people behave this way and that way. So, the way I say them, give them space…But when something bad has happened, you have to give them space. If they behave somehow strangely – forget it. It is normal that it happens, it doesn’t mean he is really behaving badly, it just happens.”

Jack emphasized the need to understand how the body and mind are interconnected. He went on to highlight the need for self-reliance and agency among police officers. He said, "Prepare yourselves… that if you want to be… good in your profession, if you want a good police, you should prepare… yourself… also, in very difficult and very critical situations we everybody has possibilities to develop ourselves… as mental and physical… and skills what we need. It's… I think it's everybody's responsibility… to understand it and do the best… they can."

DISCUSSION

Although all three participants provided a snapshot of the "psychological roller coaster" like life of a SWAT team officer, each officer's experiences gives us different pieces of the larger portrait.

Larry's experiences highlighted the unique burden of being a leader in a high-risk occupation. Timothy's experiences showed that any given situation might have lingering effects on one's psychological health in the form of fluid views on personal safety and malleable perceptions on how the world operates. Jack's story provided anecdotal evidence that certain techniques do in fact work on buffering and reversing the effects of critical incidents on law enforcement officers' psychological health.

Based on the findings that we discussed in this chapter, it is evident that techniques developed to manage high stress of SWAT work needs to be customized to officers' needs. For instance, SWAT roles differ in the types of responsibilities associated with them. Due to added responsibilities inherent with their work, officers in leadership roles may have different techniques that are more suitable for them compared to officers in positions that may not be as demanding. Further research needs to be conducted with this population to ensure that evidence-based strategies are being implemented in police organizations. Since various characteristics of SWAT work deviate from general patrol duties, it is ideal that resources are allocated towards techniques and interventions that are scientifically tested and proven to be effective with this specific population. Particularly, future studies should consider larger sample sizes to ensure that nuances of SWAT experiences are considered during development and assessment stages of stress management interventions.

Psycho-education about stress and trauma could also be more pervasive in police training curricula. It may often be the case that officers feel weary engaging in help-seeking behavior for stress-related issues for reasons described by the three officers, including perceived stigma. Embedding psycho-education about stress, trauma, and resilience in police training curricula is likely to reach a greater number of individuals. This approach is also likely to encourage officers to learn more about prevention and resilience techniques in a manner that may be more innocuous and comfortable to officers who are particularly concerned with help-seeking related stigma. An added benefit of this approach is that it allows officers access to this psycho-educational information prior to severe and repeated exposure to operational and organizational stress, potentially preventing stress-related issues from developing. SWAT officers dedicate their entire careers to protecting their communities and the civilians that comprise them, and therefore, we highly recommend that police organizations prioritize the incorporation of stress and trauma psycho-education in their training programs so that they can, in turn, assist in protecting SWAT officers.

REFERENCES

Briere, J., Kaltman, S. & Green, B. L. (2008). Accumulated childhood trauma and symptom complexity. *Journal of Traumatic Stress, 21*(2), 223–226.

Hudson, R. P. (1997). What is the future of SWAT in law enforcement? *The Tactical Edge*, *15*(4), 18-21.

Yehuda, R., Kahana, B., Schmeidler, J., Southwick, S. M., Wilson, S., & Giller, E. L. (1995). Impact of cumulative lifetime trauma and recent stress on current posttraumatic stress disorder symptoms in Holocaust survivors. *American Journal of Psychiatry*, *152*(12), 1815-1818.

EPILOGUE

Police officers are often confronted with dangerous situations in the line of duty. At the time of their admission into the police academy officers are in fact advised that working as a police officer is a difficult and challenging job and that their own survival on the street ought to be amongst their top priorities. That being said, operational law enforcement officers are aware of potential malevolent situations that they may experience at some point during the course of their careers. Amongst other things, such malicious situations may also encompass life-threatening parameters, characterized by shooting situations in the line of duty. Such situations result in traumatic experiences and, sometimes, loss (i.e., that of a partner). Police officers are trained in specialized techniques and equipment to resolve critical incident situations effectively. Notwithstanding, one of the main components that distinguish training scenarios from real life situations is the – sense of - time. Specifically, training processes give enough time for police trainees to review – along with their trainers - their own decisions, and even to get constructive feedback from both trainers and other trainees. On the other hand, an adverse incident experienced by an officer in a real life situation may require the officer to make a decision in a minuscule amount of time; that is, in a split second. The primary questions that motivated us to work on this project were: What gives survival strength to a police officer who is bleeding on the street after a fatal shooting incident? What gives strength to an officer during the moment when s/he has to find and stop a mass shooter who shoots at innocent people indiscriminately? What supports an officer to make the decision to confront and arrest a violent criminal when everybody else has tried to escape from the scene? Further, what are the symptoms of police trauma and how are these symptoms experienced by the survivor-officer after the traumatic experience?

What helps survivor-officers recover - or even adapt - to the new reality of the aftermath of trauma?

Not surprisingly, the public often present police officers as "perfect warriors" helping to instill expectations that police officers' performance in the line of duty ought to be "perfect." Consequently, any sort of negligence or human error in the line of duty is demonized by many inside and outside of the police culture.[1] The fact that many people focus their attention on officers' lack of "perfectionism" in the line of duty, leads them to misconstrue or even ignore that police officers may also be victimized in the line of duty. Furthermore, in cases where an officer makes the right decision and stops a violent criminal, it is considered by the public as "part of the job" and the officer is expected to be "back on track" right after the incident. Undeniably, research shows that police officers are more resilient than the general public. However, in this study we intended to listen to the voices of police officers who have survived traumatic experiences and, hence, examine what made them resilient and what helped them survive. In this way, we hoped to improve our knowledge in this area and to help researchers, professionals, as well as the general public in becoming aware of the reality of police officers' heroism. We hope moreover that our efforts at answering the aforementioned questions through this project will be a eulogy for those who unconditionally sacrificed - or risked - their lives in the hazards of the line of duty. In this way, we can all work towards supporting officers who have survived adverse workplace incidents. At the end of the day, officers are the ones who have been mandated to maintain peace and order, and the general public, to whom officers have sworn their allegiance, should endorse their mission.

To be continued ...

[1] Of course, we condemn cases where police officers made fatal shooting decisions due to racism or other discriminatory attitudes. In this point, we refer to vast majority of police officers who dedicate/sacrifice themselves in the line of duty to maintain peace and order and social welfare.

EDITOR'S BIOGRAPHY

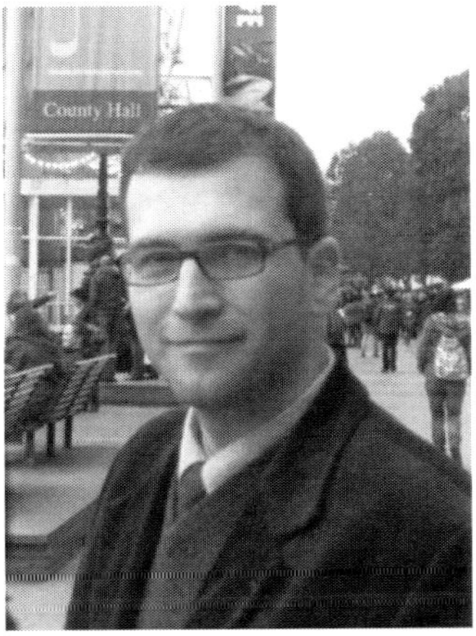

Konstantinos Papazoglou is a psychology doctoral (PhD) candidate (clinical - forensic area) and a Vanier Scholar at the University of Toronto (UofT). He is a former Police Captain of the Hellenic Police Force and he holds a master's degree in mental health counseling from New York University (NYU) as Onassis Scholar. Currently, he works with Professor Judith P. Andersen and Professor Peter I. Collins at the University of Toronto focusing his research work on stress, trauma prevention, and resilience promotion among police officers. Towards this direction he has established research collaboration with many law enforcement agencies in US, Canada, and Europe (e.g., Police Training Institute – Illinois State Police, National Police of Finland). As part of his doctoral clinical placement at the UofT-affiliated clinic, Centre for Addictions and Mental Health – Psychological Trauma Program (CAMH-PTP), he conducts assessments and provides treatment to officers suffering from trauma and stress-related issues. He has published more than 30 scholarly articles in peer-reviewed journals and book chapters. In addition, he presented his research work (more than 100 presentations) in many scientific venues (e.g., American Psychological Association, Academy of Criminal Justice Sciences, International Society for Traumatic Stress Studies) and received many awards (e.g., American Psychological Association – Criminal Justice Section Outstanding Doctoral Research Award; American Psychological Foundation – Levinson Scholarship Award; American Psychological Association – Police and Public Safety Section - Outstanding Doctoral Research Award in Police and Public Safety). Further, he conducted workshops and presented to numerous government agencies in US, Canada, and Europe (e.g., Federal Police University of Germany, Police University College of Finland, Trainer the Trainers Seminar – European Police College, Canada Department of National Defence – Research Centre, Ontario Ministry of Community Safety and Correctional Services, etc.). Konstantinos is a member of the research advisory team in Badge of Life Canada and a doctoral student representative of the American Psychological Association – Police and Public Safety Section. Moreover, he is a co-moderator of the European Medical and Psychology Experts Network (EMPEN), an official network of police health professionals established and sponsored by the European Police College (CEPOL).

AUTHORS' BIOGRAPHIES

Monica Ghabrial, MA is a PhD student in the psychology department at the University of Toronto, supervised by Dr. Judith Andersen. Her research interests include intersectionality, women's health, and sexual and ethnic/racial minority wellbeing. Monica is engaged in research that examines the unique lived experiences of Lesbian, Gay, Bisexual, Trans, and Queer people of color. This research explores the contextual discrimination and identity conflicts that this population faces, as well as the resilience they exhibit. Monica is also affiliated with Women's College Hospital, where she has investigated the effect of peer support on the wellbeing of women living with HIV.

Raquel Hudson has been involved in the strength approach and empowerment of individuals and communities, by virtue of resilience in both academia and through lived experience. Raquel holds an Honors Bachelors of Science degree in Anthropology, Psychology and Sociology, and is intrigued by the nuances of intersectionality and hope. Currently, Raquel is unpacking the "voices" of marginalized population through social work, to discover their resilience.

Shelly-Anne Li received a master's degree (MSc) in Health Research Methods at McMaster University, and is currently a PhD student studying Health Systems Research at University of Toronto. She has training and expertise in qualitative and mixed methods research, and is currently serving as a qualitative research consultant for various research projects. Extending beyond qualitative research, she has experience in leading randomized

controlled trials, designing and implementing multi-national studies, and conducting systematic reviews.
(Email address: shellyanne.li@mail.utoronto.ca)

Marian Pitel is currently pursuing her MA in Industrial-Organizational Psychology, under the mentorship of Dr. Peter Hausdorf, at University of Guelph. Prior to her graduate work, she completed her HBSc. in the Psychology Specialist program at University of Toronto. Marian worked as a Lab Coordinator at the Health, Adaptation, Research on Trauma (HART) Lab, under the supervision of Dr. Judith Andersen, investigating variables influencing performance and wellbeing of law enforcement officers. She has presented research at several conferences, including APA and ACJS, and co-authored one published peer-reviewed article. Marian is looking forward to continuing her work as a researcher-practitioner specializing in occupational health and performance.

Negin Sohbati holds an Honours Bachelor of Science from the University of Toronto (U of T). Her degree consists of a double major in Psychology and Criminology, and a minor in Sociology. She is currently a graduate student at U of T's Ontario Institute for Studies in Education (OISE), where she is pursuing a Master of Teaching. During her undergraduate career, Negin served as a senior research assistant and later, lab manager at the HART (Health Adaptation Research on Trauma) lab (2013-2016). Negin was heavily involved with research aimed at understanding the challenges of police work with the ultimate goal of improving job performance. At present, Negin is interested in exploring exceptionality in human learning. She aims to design interventions and assistive technology for specific academic skill deficits.

Peter Tam is an adjunct professor at John Jay College of Criminal Justice. His primary research interests include policing training, use of force, and motivation in becoming a police officer. He holds a master's degree from the City University of New York, John Jay College of Criminal Justice and Hunter College. He is also a 19-year veteran sergeant with the New York City Police Department currently assigned to the Office of the Commanding Officer, Police Academy. Previous law enforcement assignments include the Office of Management Analysis and Planning and Intelligence Division.

ENDORSEMENTS

I am excited to see this book, as enhanced knowledge regarding trauma exposure and resilience specifically among law enforcement officers is sorely needed. The uniqueness of the police occupation means that research findings from other trauma-exposed groups cannot be generalized to this population. That is, officers can expect to experience not only hundreds of potentially traumatic incidents throughout their careers, but these events entail many different types of traumas as well. The least commonly experienced trauma types are often the most difficult for officers to cope with during their careers. Importantly, the authors delve into this understudied aspect of the police officer experience. I am confident this book will be highly valued by criminal justice professionals, researchers, and clinicians alike.

Dr. Brian Chopko, PhD, CRC, PC,
Associate Professor of Criminology and Justice Studies,
Department of Sociology, Kent State University,
North Canton, Ohio, USA

"Traumatic stress within the policing environment is a real injury. Left untreated, it can lead to disastrous consequences for the member, their loved ones and co-workers.

For those members who suffer from operational stress injuries, including post-traumatic stress, depression, and anxiety, suicide ideation, as well as the perplexities surrounding moral injury insight through the compilation of information contained within this book will prove invaluable.

In addition, academics, treating professionals, organizations that provide insurance coverage, along with police service leadership and Human Resources professionals within policing agencies will certainly gain insight via the individual accounts and insightful research that has been accomplished in this qualitative analysis. We must remember that police personnel, like the public they serve are human after all. That members who suffer are not alone. That "Real Hero's call for back-up". That there are indeed "Strength in Numbers" when it comes to understanding that your own journey is similar to many others who are suffering. That we are truly "Hero's in Life…Not Death."

Sgt. William Rusk B.A., Executive Director,
Badge of Life Canada, Ottawa, Ontario, Canada

Papazoglou's book brings a welcomed individual, yet research-based, angle to the impact of exposure to unprecedented trauma on police officers' lives. I am confident that the book will help professionals who work with police officers to better understand the multi-faceted trauma often experienced, but not always talked about publically. The book also addresses the other side of trauma: recovery and the importance of developing evidence-based interventions in resilience promotion among police. The book is therefore essential reading to all those who strive to increase well-being of police officers.

Dr. Mari Koskelainen, Clinical Psychologist (DClinPsych)
Police University College of Finland, Tampere, Finland

INDEX

A

B

C

D

E

F

R

S

T

V

W